The Big Book of Kamasutra Sex Positions

The Beginner's Guide To Learn techniques for incredible lovemaking, transform Your Sex Life and improve intimacy in your relationship

By Susan Humphrey

Copyright ©2020 By Jamie Press
All rights reserved.
No part of this guide may be reproduced in any form without permission in writing from the publisher except in the case of brief quotations embodied in critical articles or reviews.

Legal & Disclaimer
The information contained in this book and its contents is not designed to replace or take the place of any form of medical or professional advice; and is not meant to replace the need for independent medical, financial, legal or other professional advice or services, as may be required. The content and information in this book has been provided for educational and entertainment purposes only.

The content and information contained in this book has been compiled from sources deemed reliable, and it is accurate to the best of the Author's knowledge, information and belief. However, the Author cannot guarantee its accuracy and validity and cannot be held liable for any errors and/or omissions. Further, changes are periodically made to this book as and when needed. Where appropriate and/or necessary, you must consult a professional (including but not limited to your doctor, attorney, financial advisor or such other professional advisor) before using any of the suggested remedies, techniques, or information in this book.

Table of Content

Introduction 1
Chapter 1 What is Kamasutra? 2
   History 4

Chapter 2 Sexual Compatibility 7
   Learning To Make Love 9

Chapter 3 Intimacy 13
   Becoming divine in the flesh 13
   The power and sweetness 15
   Techniques utilized 16
   Sessions utilized 16
   Suggestive Health 17
   Seven signs of sensual health 17

Chapter 4 Sex Toys for Couples 18
   Vibrating panties 18
   Vibrating Wand 18
   Cock Ring 18
   Butt Plugs or Anal Beads 19
   Feather Tickler 19
   Bondage Straps 19
   Blind Folds 20
   Hand Cuffs or Rope 20
   Sex Swing 20
   Girth Enhancers 21
   Panties with Handles 21
   Nipple Clamps 21
   "Hot Seats" or Sex Chairs 21
   Oral Sex Stimulators 21
   Electric Stimulation Toys 22

Chapter 5 Oral Sex Techniques 23

Chapter 6 Anal sex 35
Your First Time 35
Kama Sutra Positions for Anal Sex 37
Oral With Anal Stimulation 37
The Curled Angel 37
The Clip 37
The Snake 38
Pegging 38
The Curled Angel 39
Double Decker 39
Rocking Horse 39
Reverse Cowgirl 39
Doggy Style 40
Glowing Triangle 40
Reclining Lotus 40
Afternoon Delight 41
The Amazon 41
The Basket 41

Chapter 7 Pre-love Game. Secrets 42
Unique Prelude 42

Chapter 8 Positions Of Kamasutra 51

Chapter 9 Some Helpful Exercises 70
Breathing 70
Re-birthing breathing 71
Exercises to increase male orgasmic control 73
Kegels – strengthening the Yoni 74
Exercise for better sex 74
Yoga 75
The Chair 76
The Squat 76
The Cobra 77
Pranayama breathing 77
Conclusion 79

Introduction

If you are relatively new to sex and you are looking for information, tips, and sex positions, this book will give you everything you need and more. By opening up this book, you have already taken the first step in preparing yourself for your new sex life. By informing yourself as much as you can, you will ensure you are as prepared as possible so that you will be able to experience as much pleasure as you can. At the end of the day, sex is about pleasure, and knowing how best to please yourself and your sexual partners will keep them coming back to you again and again. You are going to thank yourself for having picked up this book.

The first topic we are going to discuss is what you can expect to learn through reading this book. While you will definitely learn new sex positions for every type of sexual relationship you may find yourself in (from intimate to adventurous), you will also learn so much more than that. Having sex is about more than just the positions in which you do it, so we are going to spend ample time in this book talking about the other components of a sexual relationship. These additional components include how to decide if you are sexually compatible with someone, how best to achieve orgasm for both women and men, and how to achieve and maintain intimacy. We will also look at some extra topics that can spice up your sex life when you are ready. These include sex toys, dirty talk, and any sexual fantasies you have.

Many beginner-focused sex books will begin with complete basics- beginner sex positions like missionary or cowgirl, basic tips for reaching orgasm, and basic tips like how to have shower sex safely. I recognize that you likely already know what missionary is, how to have shower sex (from seeing it in the movies), and how to give yourself an orgasm. We are going to graze over these beginner tips but spend more time on the things that will prove most useful to you in the bedroom. I will not insult you by spending 50% of the book on explaining the missionary position in great detail, but instead, I will teach you variations and new things to try once you have mastered missionary.

Read this book with an open mind and a willingness to learn. You will gain lots of new information in these pages, and it may seem overwhelming at first. The good news is, you can always flip back to any section and read it again if you forget some of the details.

Chapter 1 What is Kamasutra?

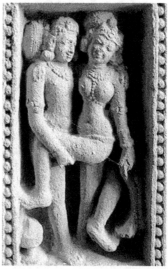

Well, you are right that it relates to sex, but that is not really the entire truth. Kamasutra is a type of romancing and getting intimate with your partner that reaches a realm completely outside of sex to make sex more interesting and more intense. While the term relies heavily on sexual positions in today's age, it still revolves around the idea that humans are inherently sexual creatures, and to staunch that sexuality is inhumane and cruel to our bodies. It brings sex out of the bedroom, and into the rest of the world in a way that makes it feel discreet and yet oh so naughty at the same time.

If you are a shy person and feel that you would not be able to do anything sexual in public, do not worry. You are most likely not going to go for a quick shag in the park. (Unless that is something you are into, though you could run into some serious legal issues if you are caught) Most of the sexuality out in your public life relies on gestures and body language, minute and subtle touches, and communication to drive the mind wild. You could be preparing your partner for the bedroom, and the people around you could have no idea what you are doing, or that you are even doing anything. That is the wonderful thing about Kamasutra. You can do all the dirty things you could imagine, and no one else than your partner would be the wiser.

Origin of the Term

This is actually an ancient Hindu term. Interesting fact. A lot of people see the Hindi people like Muslims; chaste, modest human beings who deny their sexual desires. It is actually quite the opposite. Hindi people are very sexual people. They embrace human nature, thinking it is a crime to do otherwise. If you have ever seen a Bollywood film, you will realize that the Hindi women dress very provocatively, just in a different manner than a lot of Judo-Christian women do.

Take a look at the traditional clothing that women from India wear. They often keep their midriffs exposed, and wear skirts that are at an angle to show more of one leg than the other. Their tops are often just high enough to keep from exposing their breasts, while still allowing a little room for the imagination. They wear veils that accentuate their long hair, rather than hide it. They are often adorned with jewels and other shiny objects. This is to show the natural beauty of a woman, rather than cover it up, while still keeping enough hidden to give the air of mystery and excitement. That is what Kamasutra is about. Being open with your sexual nature, but not too much so that you feel excited about the options the night can hold.

Even the men in Hindi culture dress fairly provocatively. They often wear silk shirts that are unbuttoned at the top few buttons, and loose, flowing pants that give the allusion of broadness. Their clothes are designed to allure women of their culture. Everything about the Hindi culture is beautiful, open, and gives the air of sexuality.

So it only makes sense that the term originated from one of the first cultures to embrace sexuality. It comes from the Hindi terms Kama and Sutra. Sutra is translated to mean a line, or a connection holding things together. Kama is more in depth than that, as it is one of the four goals in Hindi life. It is the third goal, the goal of sexual desire, and pleasure.

Outside the Sex

The original Kama Sutra was written sometime in the second century CE. It has since been adapted far beyond the origins, to nearly become a sex manual for people who want to go the distance but are not quite sure how. However, what the newer texts fail to realize is that it goes further than sex. You need more than a manual of positions to spice up your love life because eventually, you are going to have tried all of the positions, and then you will end up back to square one.

It is about finding a balance between your love life, and your professional life. About creating a connection between the two so that it becomes easier to transit into your love life from your professional life. You have to make sure that you are finding the balance, not just trying the new sex positions. Kamasutra is almost a way of life. Not just another category of sex in porn.

Once you learn that it is not just about the body, but also about the mind, you will find that it is a lot easier to get things going. You will see that not only has your sex life increased; your libido will rise as well. You will want to come home to your partner and ravage their bodies, and the mental connection that you will begin to feel with them will make it even better.

So there you have it. A quick run-down of what Kamasutra is. The more you understand it, the easier it will be to master it.

History

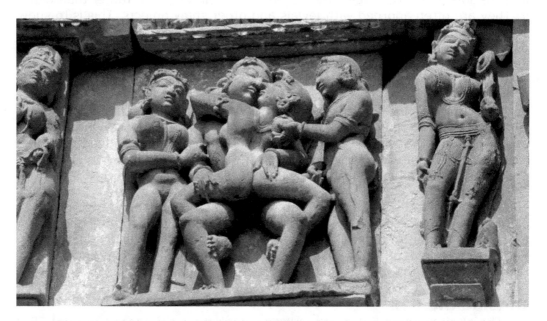

The history of the Kama Sutra is a long one. It's one of the world's eldest books about pleasure and physical living. There is no solitary author of the text, but it was initially assembled in the third century by Vatsyayana, an Indian sage who lived in the northern part of India. He claimed to be a monk practicing celibacy, and his work in amassing the sexual information of the ages was a way for him to meditate and contemplate the deity. Written in a complex form of Sanskrit, the Kama Sutra is the only remaining text of that era of early Indian history.

In scholarly circles, it's been widely consulted by scholars to determine the social mores and understand the society of that time period. The title of the text translates to a treatise on pleasure. Far more complex than just a listing of the contortionist positions, the Kama Sutra is a all-inclusive handbook of living for the good of life. Although the central character of this work is a man-about-town, the text was written to be read by and provide detailed information for both men and women.

The topics explored include social concepts, society, sexual union, the acquisition of a wife, about the wife, about the wives of other men, about courtesans, and on the ways to attract others to yourself.

In terms of finding a mate, the Kama Sutra counsels on whether to think about someone from childhood friends or fellow students. It provides diagrams that classify female and male physical types and the compatibility they will have with their lover's body. It teaches varieties of kissing, embracing, biting, scratching, oral sex, and intercourse that are elaborate. The text also has instructions on extramarital relationships, including the wives of other men, and has many pages on how to seduce and extort the courtesan.

Some refer to this book as the marriage manual, but it's a far cry from the monogamous and dutiful bindings of marriage that Westerns produced as a part of advice for couples. One of the central figures of the book is the courtesan, who must master and practice a variety of arts in order to learn how to please and coerce a man. What is unique about Kama Sutra is that maintains focus on creating pleasure for the woman, too.

Kama Sutra is the original study of sexuality, and so it became the focal point of all proceeding books, including the fifteenth century Ananga-Ranga, which was a revised version that built upon the Vatsyayana's basic beliefs. Yet due to the complex and inaccessible style of Sanskrit in which it was written, the Kama Sutra fell into obscurity for many centuries. Scholars of Sanskrit and ancient Indian did not consult it often. It wasn't until the late nineteenth century that the Kama Sutra began to resume its popularity in Indian.

The resurgence came about after the 1870's when Sir Richard Burton, a noted linguist and Arabic translator, worked with his collaborators to produce a translation of the Ananga-Ranga. When they were pursuing references to the Vatsyayana, they were led back to the Kama Sutra and an English version was produced. Burton's persistence in having this book translated so that Western readers could read it, and the interest the text generated in Indian and abroad, led to a proliferation of translations and versions of this original book.

Because of this, for many centuries the Ananga-Ranga superseded the Kama Sutra in being the text of choice to look at for knowledge about sexual pleasure. The writing of this book was ordered by the nobleman Ladakhana for one of the Lodi Dynasty's monarch. This family was a powerful part of Delhi Sultanate, who ruled over the northern part of India before the Mughal Dynasty took over. The author of the Ananga-Ranga, Kalyanamalla was a Hindu poet who referred back to the Kama Sutra heavily in order to prepare his text.

He wrote in an accessible Sanskrit style, and the royal Muslim patronage made sure that the text was circulated around the feudal Muslim kingdoms. Accounts of the Ananga-Ranga now appear in the Persian, Arabic, and Urdu cultures.

The Ananga-Ranga opens with a dedication to Ladakhana, the patron of the text, and contains prescription advice for married couples, and their conduct both socially and sexually. It starts with a detailed description of the woman's body and includes centers of passions, classifications of body types, erogenous zones, and timeliness of their sexual pleasures. Compatibility and classification of men and women by their genital size was explored in numerous combinations and to their degree of passion. Many scholars speculated that Kalyanamalla resided in more sexist civilization than the earlier writers. The noted that Kalyanamalla deviated from the other writers by neglecting to provide normative advice for producing a woman's pleasure, such as the use of fingers, that the other texts reinforce many times. The title of the book, Ananga-Ranga, has been translated to Stage of the Bodiless One, Theatre of the Love God, and The Hindu Art of Love, amongst many others.

As part of the romanticism of colonial rule, Europeans looked for Eastern texts to bring ancient wisdom to their modern world. However, the Orientalist engagement in the Ananga-Ranga led to the text's decreased relevance, and the importance of the previous Kama Sutra. Burton's experience residing in India as part of the British army and his allure with sexual practices, especially those of the Oriental societies, coupled with his desire to bring the knowledge and attention to his peers, led to his interest in the cannon of sexual knowledge that was preserved by the Sanskrit texts.

Because of the seeming popularity of the Ananga-Ranga among many Sanskrit specialists, it was only natural for it to be the text of choice for Burton's purpose. When he reviewed translations, though, he made note of the references that were made to the Vatsyayana. He believed that the earlier text, the Kama Sutra, was a far more foundational piece of work, and requested that a copy be located. Because of its neglect over the centuries, the Kama Sutra only existed in parts. The text had to be remade from Sanskrit manuscript library collections across the Princely States and Indian. Once it was translated into English, its popularity grew, and Indian scholars set aside the Ananga-Ranga with some new interest in the Kama Sutra.

Chapter 2 Sexual Compatibility

Sexual compatibility between people means that they share the same beliefs, values, preferences, desires, and expectations related to sex. This can include things like what sex acts you prefer the most, your level of sex drive, the type of sex you wish to have, including any fetishes, and so on. For example, if you have a very high sex drive, meaning that you need and expect to have sex every single day, you will be sexually compatible with someone who also has a high sex drive. If you were in a sexual relationship with someone who had a very low sex drive, this would be incompatible as you would likely become frustrated by their low need for frequent sex. Another example is if you desire a lot of oral sex and you require this in order to become fully aroused during sex, you would be sexually compatible with someone who also enjoys oral sex, especially giving it. If you were with someone who did not feel comfortable with oral sex at all, this would not make for a sexually compatible match.

Your preferences and values do not have to be exactly the same as the person you are in a sexual relationship with, but they must be able to fit together (like yin and yang) in order for a sexual relationship to be compatible. An example of this is if you enjoy slow and tender sex, but your partner enjoys rough sex. This could mean that you are sexually incompatible, but it could also work if you are both able to meet in the middle. You could start off by having slow and tender foreplay while your arousal builds, and when you are both ready for penetration, the sex can begin to lead towards a rougher style. As long as both people are comfortable with this, this sexual relationship could work.

Why is it Important?

Sexual compatibility is important when it comes to orgasm. Being sexually compatible is quite necessary for orgasm and even to find pleasure in general.

When it comes to kinks and fetishes, sexual compatibility is quite important. For example, BDSM, including dominance and submission. If you have one partner who is sexually dominant and the other who prefers submission, this works out very well. If, however, you prefer dominance and so does your partner or if both prefer submission, you may have some trouble reaching a place of agreement when it comes to your sexual encounters. The person who is dominant will not usually become turned on by being told what to do, and the person who is submissive will usually not be too excited by telling someone else what to do. While these can work on a spectrum and people can enjoy a bit of both, many people are either dominant or submissive.

If you are a person who defines themselves as either a strict dominant or a strict submissive sexual partner, you will likely communicate this quite early on in your encounters with a person. You may even communicate this before you have sex with them. This is a good idea if you have strict preferences when it comes to sex. You do not want to spend time getting to know someone who you will not be sexually compatible with for the reason that you are both unable to compromise. There are times when you will be unable to compromise in order to make yourself fit with another person sexually. This is completely alright, as sex is about pleasure. You want to make sure both you and the other person are pleased, so being communicative about your sexual preferences and values will be beneficial for everyone.

How to Determine if You are Sexually Compatible With Someone

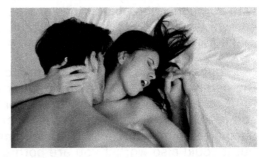

Communication is a big element of sexual compatibility. Determining if you are sexually compatible with someone relies largely on communication. By communicating your personal desires and values, you are able to see if these fit with another person's desires and values. Even if these are not the same, you can communicate about whether these are able to work together in harmony or not. If not, you are better for having communicated this instead of finding out while already in bed with that person.

This conversation can be had when you begin speaking to someone for the first time if you meet on a dating website or application where you think sex will ensue. This can be had when the sexual tension begins to build with someone whom you have been on a few dates with. This could also happen when you determine that you and this person would like to sleep together before you begin engaging in sex. Any of these times is the right time for this conversation, as you want to ensure that you are determining sexual compatibility before you begin having sex with someone. Imagine getting aroused and excited as you began kissing and touching each other, only to find out that you are both strictly dominant or that this person requires you to lick their feet when you have a fear of feet. It is best to avoid this type of situation by clearly communicating your sexual needs well in advance.

In a relationship, sexual compatibility can build over time. The first time you have sex with someone, you may be unsure if you are sexually compatible with them. As long as you both communicate and determine that there is nothing leading you to believe that you are completely incompatible. You can then allow your sexual compatibility to build as you continue your sexual relationship with each other.

It is also possible to explore your sexual compatibility with someone. If there is nothing that makes you incompatible initially, then you can explore a sexual relationship with this person. Over time, you will learn each other's bodies and how to please each other. In this way, your sexual compatibility can grow. You may find that there are things that you want to explore together or new things that you want to try with each other. As long as you both continue to communicate with each other, you can continuously determine sexual compatibility at every stage of your sexual relationship.

Learning To Make Love

When you are beginning to make love for the first number of times, you may feel awkward, wondering what positions you should do or what the other person may prefer. You may feel pressure to perform or to please your partner better than they've ever been pleased before. All of these thoughts are normal, but it is rare that a person will be an expert the first time or even the first ten times they do something new. The great thing about sex, though, is that it is a natural act for humans to engage in, which means there will be some amount of innate knowledge you will have about how to conduct yourself in a sexual encounter. Keeping that in mind, you will need to be able to trust yourself and your body in order to make the most of your first several sexual experiences.

Things to Know for Your First Time

There are some things that you must be aware of when it comes time for your first sexual encounter. Following the point that was just made above, the first thing to know is to trust yourself! At the most basic level, humans are animals. Just like any other animal, we are meant to have sex. This means that sex comes wired into our DNA and that we all have some knowledge of how to conduct ourselves during sexual intercourse. This is because our body is able to take over and follow its pleasure, its arousal and its instincts. While you don't want to act like a complete animal in bed (unless you and your partner are into it), this is simply useful to keep in mind so that you can keep your nerves at bay. If you let your mind take control, it will get in the way of and inhibit this natural instinct that you came built with.

This leads us to the next things to know, which is that relaxation and being at ease will make the encounter much more enjoyable for both of you. If you are able to relax and enjoy the experience, your body will flow much smoother, and pleasure will come much easier to both you and your partner.

The next thing to note is the importance of foreplay. In case you are unsure, foreplay is any and all of the sexual activities that come before the actual act of sexual intercourse. This can include the making out and groping, the handjob or fingering as well as oral sex or anything else you engage in before penetration occurs. This part of sex is just as important as the rest of sex because this is when you become aroused and let your arousal build before beginning penetration. It is during this time that you are able to explore each other's bodies and figure out where the other person likes to be touched the most.

Communication is the final thing to note for the first time. It may seem like there is an expectation to pretend like you know exactly what you are doing and that you have done it a thousand times before, but this is untrue. No matter who your partner is, they will be happy that you communicated and made sure that they were comfortable all along the way instead of pretending like you knew exactly what they wanted. Being able to communicate in bed is more impressive than not saying anything and guessing the entire time.

Best Positions for Your First Time

We will now look at the best sex positions for your first time. With so many possible sex positions to do, it can be overwhelming trying to decide which ones to try first. In this section, I will explain and describe the best positions for you to use during your first several sexual encounters. Keep in mind as well, that many people continue to have sex in these positions well after their first time, simply because they find the most pleasure from these positions. These are by no means reserved for your first couple of sexual encounters, especially if you thoroughly enjoy them.

Missionary

The Missionary position is that classic position that you have likely heard of a thousand times. It can sometimes be referred to as the basic or the starter position. It gets a bad reputation as the most vanilla of all positions. The missionary position, however, can actually be very, very hot, and quite intense if you make it so! Here, I will explain how to perform this position and how it can give you and your partner a world of pleasure.

To start, we are going to discuss what the Missionary Position looks like. This position is achieved when the woman lies down on her back on the bed.

Then, the man lies on top of her, his face in front of hers. The man lies with his legs between the woman's, and he inserts his penis into her from the front. Lying on top of the woman, and holding his weight up with his arms, he controls the movement in and out with his hips. Now, as I said, this position can actually be very intense if you want it to be. Because the man and woman are face-to-face, this position is actually quite intimate. The intimacy of your faces being so close together as you are in as vulnerable a position as this leads to a great connection and a great amount of pleasure. You can make out with your partner during penetration in this position to make it extra sensual. If you are in a relationship and you are making love, you can look deeply into each other's eyes, wink at them every now and then or give a slight flirty smile.

When it feels good, let your partner know by breathing the words "oh yes" into their ear, whispering dirty talk to them, or bringing your mouth close to their ear so that they can hear your moaning up close. You can even nibble on their earlobe and gently kiss their sensitive neck skin or go in for a deep and emotional kiss. Missionary can be as interesting and varied as you make it.

If you are bound to missionary because of mobility or flexibility or anything of the sort, you can use these techniques to keep it fresh for you and your partner. If you are in a new relationship or having casual sex, you can penetrate in this position with your faces farther from each other, maybe kissing every now and then, and as you get more comfortable with each other, you can gradually increase the level of intimacy and emotional connection by trying some of these ways of spicing it up and watch your relationship blossom.

Doggy

The doggy style position is a favorite among men and women alike. Both women and men can get intense pleasure from this position because the angles at which their genitals come together creates harmonic pleasure.

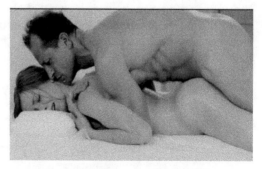

To get into this position, the woman gets on her hands and knees on the bed (or couch or floor, this position works anywhere), and the man gets on his knees behind her, both of them facing the same direction. He will then enter her from behind. The man can control the depth and speed of penetration in this position. He thrusts his hips and can control the pace in this way. He grabs onto her hips for a stronger thrust and pulls her body towards his if she wants him to thrust deeper.

Doggy style is a position that women can get a lot of pleasure from. It is no surprise it is most often the favorite position among young people of both genders. Because of the curve of the man's erect penis and the angle at which it enters into the woman's vagina, it is very likely that her G-spot will be stimulated with each thrust. This G-spot stimulation means that it will be very likely that she will reach an orgasm from penetration. G spot stimulation can make a woman feel such intense full-body pleasure for quite a long time before she actually reaches an orgasm. Hitting her G-spot will continue to feel amazing for both the woman and man until finally, one or both of them cannot wait any longer and ultimate pleasure is reached.

Cowgirl

The next position that we will look at is the Cowgirl position. As you probably already know, it is quite a bit harder for a woman to reach an orgasm from penetration than it is for a man. Therefore, it is important to be aware of which positions are able to optimize female pleasure. If your female partner has trouble reaching orgasm from penetrative sex alone, this position is one that can lead her to feel great pleasure and reach orgasm more easily than many other positions. The Cowgirl position is similar to The Missionary Position, in that both people are lying down with their faces just inches from each other. With Cowgirl, however, the woman is on top, and she is straddling the man.

To get into this position, the man will lie on the bed on his back, and the woman will straddle his waist. He can insert his penis into her from here. With the woman on top, she can control the angle of the man's penis inside of her by gliding and moving her hips in the direction and motion that feels the best for her. She can continue to move in the direction and spot that feels the best in order to reach orgasm.

If she wishes, she can sit her body upright and move up and down on the man in this position instead of lying her upper body onto her partner. In this way, this position can be as intimate or not as you wish.

Chapter 3 Intimacy

This is probably the most interesting chapter of the Kama Sutra to most of us in the West, as it concerns sexual intimacy. As I've been telling you throughout, the Kama Sutra's approach to pleasure is about pulling the disparate threads of life together, to form a pleasurable whole. Sex is at the center of that, as humanity's highest expression of earthly pleasure, but it's accompanied by a plethora of spiritual and practical life recommendations that support it.

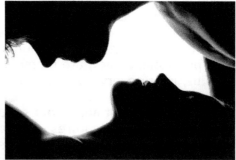

This chapter is the one most of us are most intensely interested in, so I've given it as thorough a treatment as possible here, hoping that the recommendations of the Kama Sutra and is prescriptions concerning your sexuality will help to support the re-ignition of the flame of desire between you and your partner. Following these prescriptions in context (with the rest of what I'm offering in this book in mind), you'll find that they're much more satisfying and supportive of your experience of love with your partner than they are in isolation. Life is a broad combination of factors that add up to a whole. All these factors don't exist in a vacuum. The universe, being a dynamic engine consisting of apparently opposite tensions and almost limitless variety, is the model of life itself. This can serve as the model of your lives together. Life's variety can't be segmented off and boxed into categories that isolate one of its features from all the others. The bits and pieces of our lives are not bits and pieces at all – they're dynamically interconnected, just as the universe itself is and as we all are with one another. Your romantic relationship, therefore, is designed to be the exemplar of a greater reality; a microcosm of reality itself. So, consider this chapter preparatory. What I'm sharing with you here is a Westernized interpretation of Kama Sutra, which will prepare you and your partner to explore your sexuality with eyes that see its sacred nature, as well as your own sacredness.

Becoming divine in the flesh

Implicit in Kama Sutra is an invitation to all lovers to join in the cosmic dance. Whether we're aware or not, the joining of loving bodies in physical demonstrations of desire is a sacred act. Regardless of the nature of the act, to love physically is to participate in the divine dance. In making love with one another, we weave ourselves into the universe and come part of its integral whole. We help to hold it together.

If that sounds like a big responsibility, it's because you've never approached your sexuality from this standpoint before. When you actually undertake to do so, the whole thing becomes a lot less daunting. It just feels right. That's because it is.

Your sexuality and living it out in a wholesome, joyful way is part of the divine plan and an important component of cosmic harmony. When the energy that passes between two people is intense and incarnated through acts of physical intimacy, you draw closer to the divine without even understanding that's the case. The many moments of our live we spend in sexual congress, or in physical intimacy, are moments in which we lift the veil that conceals from us, in our everyday lives, the true nature of godhead.

We are part of it and in our sexuality, we are living out our most extravagantly divine natures. This is an awesome thought I'd like readers to make special note of. In fact, there's an exercise, I would encourage you all to try. Take off your clothes. Now, go look at yourself in a full length mirror. Take the time to really look at yourself, to move your arms and legs, to smile at yourself and to examine the wonder of your beautiful, human body.

There may be some bumps, lumps, zig zags and ripples we look at and would prefer not to see. Every one of those presumed imperfections, though, is a wonderful and unique story about the incredibly individual nature of our bodies. We all have these unpredictable, ripply, lumpy, bumpy bodies. They share some common features. But our bodies are also specifically us. The human body is a tale of life and all it entails – the good, the bad, the challenging and the terrifying. Our bodies are like passports, stamped by our days and years with the experiences we've had, the adventures we've survived and the imprints of thousands of those who have come before us, making us who we are. We are incredibly complex beings and this is reflected in the wondrous human body.

Looking at your physical self and seeing yourself for what you are is a doorway to seeing others in the same, expansive and wonderstruck way. Your body isn't a crackerjack box. It's you. It's what people see and say, "There's thingamabob!" It's your calling card and your way of involving yourself in the day to day life of the world around you. Without it, you'd be a disembodied, amorphous Casper the Friendly Ghost, drifting about unnoticed (or perhaps scaring the living crap out of people). What I'm saying is simple – your body is what makes you human. All of it. Even the parts you don't particularly care for. Your body is your story.

The first and most important part of loving another person as they are, is loving yourself. When you can behold yourself nude and vulnerable, you'll be able to see your partner more compassionately, less judgmentally and more appreciatively. Now get ready to put that renewed vision of love to good use, as we explore the Kama Sutra's gifts to sexuality.

Your flesh is what the divine works with. God has no hands but ours. You are an instrument of the divine in the cosmos, working to hold together and uplift the harmonious interplay and balance of the universe. When the two become one, all is whole. When you love, the music of the spheres is heard, as the stuff of Creation is knit together again and sustained. Love is divine and making love as a co-creation of the universe, through every touch, every sigh and every movement of our bodies together, makes of us god's partners. Through our sexual natures, we come as close to the divine order in the cosmos as we may, as mere human beings. We become divine.

Sacred Intimacy is certifiably not a single procedure or activity. It is an approach of welcoming the aggregate of your body - physical, mental, emotional, spiritual, sexual - into the session. Any bodywork by its nature is a sensual encounter, engaging your body's largest organ - the skin.

The skin has covered an average of 22 square feet on an adult. This amazing surface is furnished with endless scrumptious means of experiencing the world. Too often, nonetheless, we allow ourselves to ignore the sexual nearness of our skin. We push aside its story, questioning its intensity. We allow its receptivity to be dull, unaware of its plausibility.

I feel that my activity as a Sacred Intimate is to assist you with waking up - wake up to be more present, more powerful, and more aware in this body. At this moment. With whatever challenges or blessings exist.

The power and sweetness

The power and sweetness of a man's touch are of vital importance to my background as a gay man. I am equally aware of how oblivious or careless touch can reinforce, rather than help release, patterns of bluntness or shame that a man may bring to a bodywork session. Also, this sort of touch can also fail to acknowledge completely the delight and pleasure that can arise during the session.

My training in massage, Mariel healing (energy work similar to Reiki), and Vipassana Buddhist meditation all add to my being awake and intuitively present with my customers. Attending many sorts of workshops over many years with the Body Electric School and other explorations of spirituality and sexuality have given me a feeling of spontaneity, miracle, and fun in guiding men through their sessions.

The blessings and challenges of our lives are as varied as our bodies. Those of us who don't fit easily into prohibited social norms will, in general, experience the limits of these posts of experience regularly. Sacred Intimate work acknowledges and values this variety, allowing for many various types of sessions and encounters, using various means and intensities.

Healing and Transformation

The two pillars of my approach to Sacred Intimate work are healing and transformation. These broad ideas assist me with guiding you to the kind of session that will be generally beneficial and send them out the door with a grin.

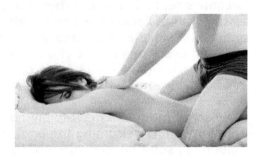

Techniques utilized

Techniques utilized can include:
- Sensual massage
- Breath of Life Massage
- Anal massage
- Breathwork
- Ritual
- Visualization

Issues that can be addressed can include:
- Letting go of old habit patterns or stories
- Fear of expressing your needs, desires
- Setting new goals
- Sexual abuse
- Boredom
- Addiction
- Isolation
- Fears related to intimacy
- Body shame
- HIV status

or essentially rejoicing in what your identity is at this moment.

Sessions utilized

Sessions can include:
- Touching and be touched as a lover
- Eye-gazing and shared breathwork
- Instruction and/or witnessing of self-pleasuring
- Creating rituals to honor your body, life, work, milestones
- Working with couples to teach intimacy and pleasure aptitudes and affirm commitment

- Dying practice to release troubles and appreciate what your identity is at present
- Roleplay to act out fantasies.
- Gentle body contact and snuggling to encounter warmth and comfort

Suggestive Health

Hardly any of us had a suggestive mentor when we were youthful - somebody who knew and cared for their own body intimately and shared that information with us lovingly and capably. Hardly any, of us think of our sensual lives in a wholistic, regenerative and positive way - it is rather a progression of somewhat-associated snapshots of "getting a few," "getting enough" or "getting off" with a fantasy tossed in once in a while for flavor.

Sacred Intimacy is an invitation to recuperate this missing mentoring, to find the obscure parts of yourself and reveal another and exciting segment of your health.

Here are a lot of brilliant markers of suggestive health, formulated by Jack Morin in his book "The Erotic Mind." They outline a way of thinking about this part of ourselves in a refreshing, non-judgmental and open way

Seven signs of sensual health

1. The erotically healthy individual builds up a clear arrangement of ethical values that have intrinsic personal meaning
2. Erotically healthy individuals establish safe parameters within which to release themselves.
3. Erotically healthy individuals perceive that sexual fantasies and behaviors operate in two separate yet interrelated circles.
4. Erotically healthy individuals make the most of their fantasies as well as use them to gain insights into their feelings and motivations.
5. Erotically healthy individuals who are involved with youngsters take an interest in their sexual improvement, especially the advancement and nurturance of positive, self-affirming attitudes toward sex.
6. Erotically healthy individuals accept and appreciate their sexual uniqueness rather than fearing or fighting it.
7. Erotically healthy individuals appreciate decent sexual variety in others as well as in themselves.

Chapter 4 Sex Toys for Couples

Sex toys and tools are a fun addition to enhance your sex life. The following are a variety of toys and tools that can be used by couples to spice up the bedroom life. These toys can be used simply for fun, or as a part of role playing. Sex toys tend to increase the amount of stimulation being experienced by one or both partners, creating more explosive orgasms. They can also enhance the intimacy between lovers, as you learn what each other enjoy most.

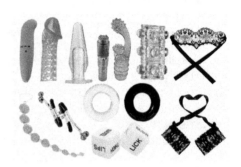

Vibrating panties

These are a fun way to encourage foreplay long before you even hit the bedroom. Vibrating panties that have a remote control feature can be worn on a date night, with the gentleman controlling the remote control. He can then turn it on and off at his own desire, having his lady at his mercy until he is ready to have his way with her. These can also be awesome if you purchase a crotchless panty variety, as they can stay on and turned on during sex to continue the stimulation throughout the encounter.

Vibrating Wand

Wands are a fun way to add pleasure to the sexual experience. You can apply as much or as little pressure as you desire, and either partner can be in control of the wand. It can be used on either partner, and doesn't have to be limited to the sex organs. To enhance the experience, you can trace your partner's inner thighs or butt with the wand while it is switched on.

Cock Ring

There are a variety of different cock rings available on the market. They are believed to assist gentlemen in lasting longer, and help make him rock hard. If you are just looking for a simple cock ring, there are a variety of silicone varieties that are stretchy and apply and remove easily. Alternatively, you can purchase a vibrating cock ring that can provide stimulation to her clitoris with each thrust, while also providing a consistent vibrate to his penis during sex.

Butt Plugs or Anal Beads

If you are into anal play, butt plugs and anal beads come in a variety of fun forms. There are butt plugs with rhinestones on them, butt plugs shaped like hooks, small ones, large ones, there are anal beads that increasingly get larger, or several same-sized ones on a string. There are several anal-play toys that can be used during vaginal penetration to create a double penetration experience for the woman. This can also be enjoyable for the man, as he can typically feel it against his penis while he penetrates her vagina, and can even make it feel tighter and more textured for him.

Floggers

There are a variety of floggers and whips that can create an enjoyable bedroom experience for those interested in a BDSM-style experience. It is important that if you use these toys, you realize that they are not intended to be used with great force, but rather with gentle but consistent force. You do not want to cause bodily harm to your lover. That being said, a good spanking with a flogger can add many levels of pleasure to your sex.

Feather Tickler

These, as well as other textured toys are excellent for stimulating the senses while having sex. They can be used in virtually any way to entice senses that aren't normally triggered during sex. For example, you can blind fold your partner and then trace their body with the feather tickler, or you can gently run it over their penis or vagina to increase blood flow to their sex organs and turn them on even more. The opportunities are endless with these types of toys.

Bondage Straps

These straps come in a variety of different shapes and sizes, and are used to help support the submissive during bondage sex moves. Some of these straps include ones to help support the tummy to keep their bum up high, ones that keep legs high, or ones that keep arms behind their back. You can find these on any number of sex toy sites that sell bondage gear.

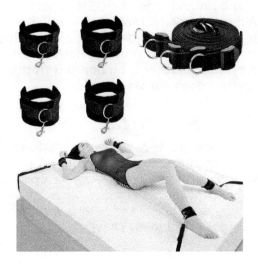

Lingerie

Believe it or not, sexy ensembles are not strictly for women to wear. Although there is a vast number of lingerie outfits for women to wear for her man, there are also many for men to wear. Adding lingerie is an incredible way to enhance sexual pleasure. You can even use lingerie to dress up as certain roles and include role playing in your intimate encounters. Some inspiration for role playing includes: doctor and patient, cop and prisoner, secretary and boss, or anything else that turns you on and helps liven up your sexy time.

Blind Folds

There is a certain level of mystery that comes with using blind folds during sex. The blind folded partner will experience increased physical awareness as they are no longer able to see what is happening to them. It enhances the excitement with each touch they experience, while also removing the element of expecting what is yet to come. When your partner is blind folded, you can add to their pleasure by using a variety of different textured items to stimulate sensitive areas on their body. (I.e. feather on the thighs, silk on the lower back, pearls on the chest, etc.)

Hand Cuffs or Rope

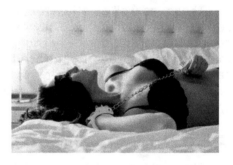

Having your partner tied down or restricted can greatly enhance their sexual pleasure. It takes away from their ability to react, almost forcing them to take anything you have to give them. It can be an exciting way to take control in the bedroom and enjoy a BDSM experience. Almost everyone has some level of desire to be tied down and have someone else take their way with them. However, make sure your partner is on board with this as you should never do something your partner does not want to do.

Sex Swing

There are several swings made specifically for sex that can deeply enhance the sexual experience. You will need to have a solid place to mount your swing, but they can create a wonderful opportunity to create a more fluid movement for penetration. Also, they generally have customizable settings so you can control the height and the way in which the person sitting in the swing is positioned. They are a wonderful addition to any intimate bedroom!

Girth Enhancers

While these aren't for everyone, they are out there. These toys are similar to cock rings, except they're longer and thicker. They generally help the gentleman last much longer, while also filling the woman up much more. They resemble dildos, except have a hole in the center where the gentleman's penis fits inside. Girth enhancers can be a fun way to change up the pace and style, and can even be a part of role playing to make it feel as though you are with someone else entirely.

Panties with Handles

There is a special type of crotchless panties available on the market that have handles on either side. These handles are wonderful for helping the gentleman gain leverage while he thrusts into the lady. Often, they are used during positions such as doggy or other positions where the lady is face-down.

Nipple Clamps

These clamps are generally set to only squeeze a certain amount and are applied to the nipples during sex. They help to stimulate other areas on the body, and increase the amount of pleasure felt by the wearer. While they are traditionally used by females, there are many males who enjoy wearing nipple clamps as well. Nipples are a very sensitive part of the body, so including them in sex can help have a full body orgasm.

"Hot Seats" or Sex Chairs

These chairs are generally little round poufs that have a dildo in the center. The dildo can be used to achieve a double-penetration experience for the female. They are generally blow-up chairs that have no sides or backings, so you can position yourself in whatever way is comfortable for you. They are easy to put up and take down, and are wonderful for anyone looking for something different and with maximum pleasure for her, if she's OK with anal.

Oral Sex Stimulators

Similar to vibrating toys, these toys feature several little tongue-shaped pieces that spin quickly to create the sensation of receiving oral pleasure. They are wonderful for couples as they can be used to stimulate the lady's clitoris during sex to increase her chances of having an orgasm. They can also be used on other areas of the body to stimulate sensations that aren't normally felt during sex, to further create a full-body experience.

Paddles

Paddles can be made from a variety of materials, including leather, wood, metal, and more. They are generally smaller, hand-held toys that look exactly how they sound: like paddles. These are used to spank your partner, and can be used anywhere on their body. The most common places include the cheeks, their bottom, and their feet. Always take care to use the tool gently, as you do not want to cause bruising or harm to your partner. This toy is not to abuse your partner, but rather to stimulate a naughty sensation. You always want to use light, but consistent pressure when you're using it. Make sure you're extra gentle if you're using it on their face, and that they approve of such things before you try. You do not want your partner to be, feel or look as though they are being abused!

Electric Stimulation Toys

These toys are a little bit pricier, but work by sending subtle but noticeable electric shocks through your partner. When used properly, they are not dangerous, and can greatly enhance the sensation of a full-body experience. They are perfect for stimulating parts of the body which are otherwise neglected during sex. You can purchase these from almost any sex store, and they can be used on either partner. They are a fun and unique addition to your sex life, if this is the type of thing you are interested in.

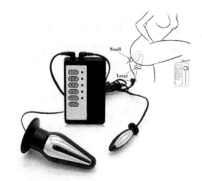

Chapter 5 Oral Sex Techniques

Oral sex starts with the main profound kiss, and proceeds with kisses everywhere throughout the body, focusing at last on the private parts. With respect to the supplier, it requires a level of the enthusiastic association since it must be finished with persistence, delicacy, affectability, and mounting however controlled energy in the event that it is to be great. Sweethearts 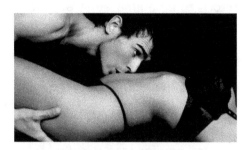 who give oral sex hesitantly and without liberality or delight make their accomplices feel regretful and narrow-minded, and excessively tense and stressed to unwind and take joy themselves.

Inappropriate, against the ethical code, and not for learned courteous fellows was the Kama Sutra's assessment of oral sex. However, that didn't prevent Vatsyayana from depicting in delicious detail precisely how a eunuch or male hireling should bow between his lord's legs and "suck the mango" or "gobble up".

From the recipient, oral sex requires trust and the certainty that accompanies being made to feel attractive. In sex, as indifferent everyday issues, it is frequently more hard to get liberality than to give it, however, the individual who surrenders totally to joy conveys oneself over to the darling, and this additionally gives a feeling of wonderment. It's a given that sexual cleanliness is of prime significance for any individual who takes part in oral sex.

Oral sex for ladies is called cunnilingus. For some ladies, cunnilingus is the most energizing of the considerable number of varieties of sex, and a delicate and skillful darling ought to have the option to make his accomplice accompany his tongue more effectively than in some other manner. A solid tricky tongue can be utilized with exactness on the clitoris without risk of causing any torment, in contrast to a finger.

Start by kissing your accomplice's face and mouth, and afterward, bit by bit work your way down her body, kissing and stroking her bosoms, tummy, and internal thighs. Flick your tongue in light fluffy kisses along the plump creases of the external labia, smoothing endlessly the pubic hair and afterward separating the labia tenderly with your fingers. Move slowly inwards with your tongue. Differ your developments as per your accomplice's reaction. Have a go at nestling, tunneling, pushing with your tongue into her vagina, sucking, long sensitive licks, and short quick flicking licks. She dislike her clitoris to be animated straightforwardly from the outset, so continue probably until she is completely stirred.

When she can confide in YOU and feel sure that you like what you are doing, she will be capable completely to give up in climax. Being 'on the detect', a man can get a unique rush from encountering so straightforwardly the euphoric impact he has on his accomplice, just as from her helplessness and trust.

Oral sex for men is called fellatio. The experience of having their penis sucked, licked and kissed is one that most men find strongly energizing. Now and again, there might be mental obstructions to survive. A few men dread being chomped during oral sex. The lady should open her mouth as wide as could be allowed, and close her lips, yet not her teeth, over the penis. Utilizing every one of the muscles in the lips and tongue will imply that the teeth should not come into contact with the penis by any means.

A few ladies are concerned that they might be stifled during fellatio. The best approach to alleviate this dread is to stay in charge: you are the person who should move while your accomplice lies still, so there is no plausibility of his pushing profound into your throat and making you choke. A few ladies consider gulping semen offensive. Obviously, there is no requirement for you to do this on the off chance that you don't wish to, yet numerous ladies do appreciate having their accomplice discharge into their mouths.

Work your way down your accomplice's body, starting with kissing his face and mouth and advancing to his privates. Be delicate, as they are profoundly touchy to torment. There are numerous methods for invigorating the penis with your lips and tongue. You can lick up and down the pole with a sensitive tongue, at that point utilize more weight and press your open lips just as your tongue against it as you rub them all over towards the head. You can lick and kiss the frenulum - the delicate spot where the glans joins the pole on the underside, which will look towards you if the man is lying on his back with an erection. You can take the leader of the penis in your mouth and suck it, stimulating it simultaneously with your tongue, and you can move your lips as far down the pole as is agreeable. At that point go here and there, sucking and squeezing with your lips and tongue.

The '69' position is alleged in light of the fact that the figures take after a couple giving each other oral sex. While numerous couples locate this a decent method for stirring one another, others think that it is hard to focus on giving and accepting such exceptional joy simultaneously. On the off chance that you are going to come in this position, it is ideal to sever from pleasuring your accomplice to dodge unintentionally gnawing the person in question. Utilize your fingers to show to your accomplice what's going on and let yourself go in the climax.

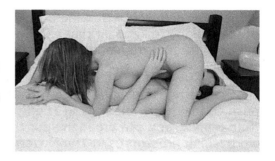

Unsatisfactory practices

Fellatio in the Kama Sutra is absolutely a method for a worker to fulfill his lord in the middle of his loving undertakings. Vatsyayana favored not to recognize that a pure and delightful lady may go down on her if he mentions that "ladies of the group of concubines" may at times enjoy somewhat oral to breathe easy.

Oral sex to die for

If you do not have (or need) a helpful eunuch or group of concubines, you'll need to manage with one another. Albeit oral is an extraordinary method to warm each other up before sex, have a go at making it your principle course instead of only a starter. Realizing that your sweetheart is focused on going all the way is an amazing sexual enhancer. At the point when you're doing the giving, make it hot, wet, and wild. If your sweetheart sees that you're cherishing it, they'll love it much more. At the point when you're in a bad way, show your thankfulness as groans, moans, and "Mmmmm"s.

Regardless of anything else, take as much time as is needed. Bother before you go in for the kill. Linger on your sweetheart's inward thighs, perineum, or pubic triangle. Invest your energy kissing, tickling, nestling, and licking. Ensure that your sweetheart is humming with desire before you apply your lips to the clitoris or penis.

Intimate Union

The following sex positions are made for exotic sessions before a log fire, love-ins in a four-publication bed, or making out in a late spring glade... or classic room. They are packed with sentiment, closeness, and soul-merging at the top of the priority list. Think tantric as opposed to torrid.

Here you can test the nose-to-nose adorableness of Butterflies in Flight, the radiantly close Singing Monkey, and the pleasures of the provocatively named Cat and Mouse Sharing a Hole. In any case, don't depend on the position alone to keep up that sentimental power; proceed with the seething eye to eye connection and fingertip strokes.

Similarly, that you'd pick the correct wine to go with a delightful dinner, choose the right sex style to go with the position, for example, profound pushing may work superbly in The Stopper-age, yet be awkward in Coitus from Behind. You can broaden your collection of sex strokes by adapting some old pushing procedures in The Movements of Sex.

Generally opened position

The lady has an unordinary measure of space to express her desire in this minor departure from the conventional man-on-top position. Since his hips are high noticeable all around instead of sticking her to the bed, she's allowed to push, granulate, and squirm as much as she needs.

Why it works

- **You alternate to lead the pack:** she pushes upward when it's her turn in control; he pushes descending when it's his.
- When she's the one making the moves, he encounters an exciting descending draw on his pole.
- You can tailor the situation to your state of mind. You can pummel your bodies against one another in wild forsake or make little, delicate developments in snapshots of heartfelt closeness.
- He doesn't put any weight on her, which is helpful if she's pregnant.

Two fishes and Swallows in affection

Attempt this pair of positions when you need prodding to develop to sex. Entrance is troublesome in Two Fishes, so you can go through it to slope the sexual pressure. At that point, when you're so tense you can't tolerate it any longer, she can move on to her back and open her legs wide in welcome.

Why they work

- Two Fishes is an extraordinary situation for bunches of skin-stroking, ass-grabbing, and profound kissing foreplay. It gives you both sufficient occasions to heat up and get your juices streaming.
- He can kick-start her excitement by slipping his hand around to stroke her labia and clitoris.
- Swallows in Love (a.k.a. the evangelist position) is a nitty-gritty man-on-top situation in which you're both allowed to focus on the in-out development of his penis.
- She can snatch his butt to impact the mood, pace, and profundity of his pushes, and rock her pelvis so as to his developments.

Parallel grasp

You both untruth straight and parallel on your sides, he envelops her with his arms as you kiss enthusiastically. He enables his hands to wander over her butt and thighs.

The snare

She shares her legs over the highest point of his in Two Fishes position. He pushes against her body without entering her.

Turning over

She turns over on to her back while he continues kissing her from the side.

Man on top He jumps over her, and she opens her legs to give him access. This is Swallows in Love. He takes his weight on his lower arms as he pushes unreservedly.

The principal act

This stance is suitably named on the grounds that it's regularly the primary position that sweethearts get into when they need classic, man-on-top sex. It's not athletic, outlandish, or masterful, yet for basic, agreeable sweetness, it can't be beaten.

Why it works

- He gets the fulfillment of pushing openly and profoundly on the grounds that her knees are raised.
- The shaft of his penis contacts her clitoris on each push, giving her significant erosion where she needs it most.
- You're very close, so the joy on your darling's face is plain to see. You can sustain off one another's excitement to drive the force of your lovemaking out of this world.
- Her hands are allowed to wander all over his body to make this position especially exotic just as sexual.

Midsection to stomach

Here and there sex should be quick and upstanding... Perhaps you're doing it in the shower, or possibly you're outside and you can't rest. Whatever your setting, Belly to Belly is a most optimized plan of attack course to infiltration, without losing the closeness of vis-à-vis, skin-on-skin contact.

Why it works

- You can move on from kissing to out and out sex in a moment or two. The promptness of your desire is a love potion for both of you.

- You don't have to strip; she just sneaks off her undies and lifts up her skirt. He at that point drops his jeans, and away you go.
- His penis enters her at an irregular edge, making a lot of invigorating erosion against her clitoris and labia.
- You can make sex feel extra-filthy by disclosing to one another your naughtiest dreams, as you are at such lacking elbow room.

Catching and Side-by-side fastening

Catching is a hot variety of the preacher position in which she traps him with her feet around his legs. To blend things up mid-session, you turn over into a one next to the other position. What's more, if you need to, you can continue rolling with the goal that she has a turn on top as well.

Why they work

If you both utilize a shaking movement in the Clasping position, she has a decent possibility of arriving at the climax. She shakes down while he shakes up.
- The Clasping position is probably the best position for nestling, embracing, snuggling, kissing, and kissing.
- Side-by-Side Clasping changes the rhythm and puts her on an increasingly equivalent premise; she can push to and from while he stays still.
- Rolling on to your sides is a decent method to temper his desire and make sex last more if Clasping is pushing his catches too rapidly

Love's combination

This is what might be compared to a cup of cocoa: warm, supporting, and soothing. He takes her in his arms, and she cuddles against him as you tenderly rock against one another. What you pass up in confounding energy you'll compensate for in closeness, sentiment, and delicacy.

Why it works
- In this position, his penis bumps her vaginal passageway or infiltrates by only a modest quantity. This is beneficial for her in light of the fact that the external third of the vagina is the part that is generally delicate to incitement.
- He gets the opportunity to show his minding side by adopting a delicate and cherishing strategy to sex.
- There's no presentation pressure on her; she can lie back and feel snuggled and secure in his arms.
- Love's Fusion encourages you to bond when you've been away from one another, or to make up after you've had a contention.

Mandarin duck

This surprising position includes some requesting leg tangles; it may not be the quickest course to entrance and climax, yet it's amusing to attempt in case you're in an innovative, trial temperament. You can generally snicker and tumble your way into a simpler position on the off chance that it turns out badly

Why it works

- The point at which his penis enters her vagina may deliver some new and inebriating sensations.
- You both appreciate the fulfillment of giving something somewhat a shot of the customary.
- You can have a great time helping out one another to get into position.
- You'll be so engrossed with making sense of which leg ought to go where that you'll leave all your sexual restraints behind.
- You're vis-à-vis, so you can appreciate each other's demeanors of delight/diversion.

Squeezing and Twining

Praise your affection in these two sincerely charged positions. You're going to be secured an energetic vis-à-vis secure in which he does the squeezing and she does the twining. So put the silk sheets on the bed, light the candles, and let the cherishing start.

Why they work

- Although he's in the predominant position, sex remains intuitive. She controls his energy by embracing his top half in her arms and encasing his base half between her legs.
- Pressing and Twining stream flawlessly into one another. There are a lot of other leg positions she can explore different avenues regarding as well, for example, moving her knee or fixing her leg.
- When he feels her heel on the rear of his leg in twining position, he realizes that she needs him more profoundly inside her.
- You can be as physically and genuinely close as you like in these positions; they're ideal for the can't-keep-your-hands-off one another phase of a relationship.

Butterflies in flight

Most well-known lady on-top positions highlight her sitting or bowing with on leg on each side of his abdomen and riding him cowgirl-style. A butterfly in Flight is increasingly delicate and alluring. She stays in control, while he gets the advantage of feeling all her erogenous zones moving tenderly down on his.

Why it works
- She can test and position herself with the goal that his penis enters her at the most suggestively fulfilling point.
- He encounters the energy of playing a latent job during sex. He's nailed somewhere around her body, and her hands and feet are over his, so it's hard for him to move.
- It's an opportunity to engage in sexual relations at a quieter pace than expected; you can both relish the unpretentious developments and sensations.
- She can propel herself all over in little, however attractive developments with her arms, legs, and center quality, utilizing his feet as a stage.

Grasping with toes
The closeness of Gripping with Toes originates from his solid savage on-each of the fours stance encasing her helplessness. Since she's half suspended with her legs around his middle, she's, for the most part, subject to him to make the moves. Supporting this difficult situation for a whole sex session relies upon whether her thigh muscles can take care of business.

"Kisses, snack, sucking of lips, fastening of bosoms, and drinking energy-charged salivation are the things that make solid love. On the off chance that you do these things, the two discharges will happen all the while, and pleasure will be finished for both of you."

Grasping with toes

Why it works
- If she has solid thigh muscles, she can give him tasty sensations by pulling herself all over on his body (consider pull-ups on an exercise center bar).
- He adores the sentiment of her legs bolted energetically around his middle.
- You can both experience the potent rush of oddity and the fulfillment of pulling off a dubious move; it is difficult to have intercourse when she's incompletely suspended.
- Her head is lower than her feet, so she gets a surge from being marginally reversed.
- Athletic positions, for example, this requires sexual collaboration. When you've taken a stab at Gripping with Toes, you'll need to push your sensual limits significantly further.

Transverse lute and Placid grasp

The mind-set is definitely not tranquil in this smaller than expected grouping. After a serious kiss lying on your sides, you both turn over by 90 degrees with the goal that she's on her back. He at that point gets her and aides her onto his prepared and willing erection.

Why they work

- In the Placid Embrace, he can enter profoundly, and she can either watch the power of his longing or recline and appreciate the ride.
- Side-by-side positions, for example, the Transverse Lute imply that both of you can lead the pack in moving, kissing, and touching.
- The Transverse Lute additionally allows you to enjoy loads of spine-shivering foreplay and get under one another's skin before he really enters.
- Moving from the Transverse Lute to the Placid Embrace makes an exciting state of mind change; she is cleared into his arms as he assumes responsibility.

The pine tree

This provocative position is alleged in light of the fact that the lady's raised legs take after the tall, exquisite trunk of a pine tree; ideal for tree-huggers all over the place. Attempt the Pine Tree when you're in the state of mind for sex that is X-appraised and hot, yet cherishing and close as well.

Why it works

- He's in a steady position that lets him control how quick and profound his developments are. Any varieties produce exciting sensations for both of you.
- Lying on her back with her legs extended straight noticeable all around makes her vibe supple and athletic, yet attractive as well.
- He gets a sensual frisson from being held under control by her legs as he enters her.
- She can fix him with a provocative look as he looks at her through her thighs.
- Her hands are allowed to delight both of you.

The fifth stance

This straightforward position is a great arousing blessing from him to her. His main responsibility is too luxurious her stripped body done with amazing touches while delicately having intercourse to her. Her activity is just to lie back and appreciate: what more could any young lady request?

Why it works

- Because he doesn't infiltrate her completely, the delicate external third of her vagina gets a large portion of the consideration.
- She can concentrate only without anyone else joy with no strain to respond.
- He encounters the rush of making her dissolve.
- It's ideal for early morning wake-up sex; you're both warm and tired, and you get a delicate yet suggestive beginning to the day.
- If his erection travels every which way, it doesn't make a difference, in light of the fact that the accentuation is on erotic touch as opposed to immovable pushing.

The developments of sex

The manner in which you granulate your pelvis, go all over or undulate your entire body can have the effect between unsurprising sex, and unstable sex that will leave you limp and wheezing. Here are some development recommendations from the Kama Sutra and The Perfumed Garden.

On the off chance that you ordinarily siphon your approach to climax with no variety in style, pace, or beat, set yourself a test, imagine you've never had intercourse and need to make sense of how to move without any preparation. Attempt each sort of development from bobbing, shaking, scouring, and hovering to squirming, shaking, crawling, and undulating; and that implies both of you. Indeed, even take a stab at remaining still for the infrequent minute during sex. In the event that you feel senseless, turn off the lights.

Stirring

This includes him taking the base of his pole immovably close by and whirling the tip of his penis along the length of her vulva. The primary feature of his visit ought to be her clitoris, utilizing to and fro flicks or firm circles, with periodic temporary re-routes to her vaginal passage, where he presses and beats his glans.

This can lead on to another prodding stroke known as Love's Tailor, in which he slips the tip of his penis a little route inside her and rubs it here and there. It is incredible for her on the grounds that, as the Kama Sutra says, a "lady's tingle is generally broad in the external piece of her vagina." Then, exactly when she's becoming acclimated to shallow in-and-out developments, he can give her the rush of the unforeseen by all of the sudden diving in the whole distance. He can differ his strokes from shallow excessively profound all through sex.

Love's bond

This is the place he infiltrates her, so the full length of his penis is inside her, at that point delays for an ecstatic most extreme entrance minute. This can lead to the well-known in-and-out movement of intercourse; he can push more than once without pulling back, which is known as Sporting of a Sparrow. The Kama Sutra says this happens "toward the finish of intercourse." To make it as animating as could be expected under the circumstances, keep the developments light, liquid, and long. Another mid-sex method to attempt includes him pulling back totally and afterward reappearing at top speed, known as giving a Blow. It's not to everybody's taste; thus, on the off chance that you attempt it, pick an agreeable situation in which you can make certain of a smooth reemergence.

A lady putting on a show of a man

Every one of the strokes so far has been for men to do on ladies, yet the jobs can undoubtedly be turned around, so she is the dynamic party. The Kama Sutra likewise portrays how she can turn around on his penis in The Top, hold him firmly in The Mare, and rock on his penis in The Swing.

Rock with me

Sex specialists regularly prescribe a shaking procedure to assist ladies with arriving at climax. She lies on her back with him on top. His careful position is significant: he needs to "enjoy some real success" on her body with the goal that the base of his penis is scouring toward her clitoris. He can accomplish this by infiltrating her, at that point shimmying up her body until he can't get any higher without his penis sneaking out. Presently you start the immensely significant shaking. As she shakes her pelvis down toward the bed, he shakes his toward the roof. This pulls a huge piece of his pole out of her. Next, she shakes her pelvis toward the roof as he shakes his toward the bed. This brings his whole penis back inside her, causing tight, sliding rubbing against her clitoris. Rehash until peak!

Singing monkey

She takes control in this agreeable yet provocative lady on-top position. It's sex at its slowest and sauciest. It's likewise an extraordinary open door for her to get him a sensual exhibition where she flaunts her body. He, in the interim, kicks back and appreciates the ride.

Why it works

Her legs are spread wide so entrance is profound and simple, and she can without much of a stretch animate her clitoris with her fingers.

She can investigate various sensations by reclining on her hands to change the point at which his penis enters her.

It's a sure and attractive situation wherein you can take as much time as is needed, recline on your hands, and value one another.

You can kiss however much you might want. Start with provisional lip and tongue contacts, and progress to an exceptional mouth-merging that flabbergasts you.

Cicada on a branch

He crawls up and takes her from behind in this smooth variation of sex from behind. You both get all the unusual sensations and advantages of back section sex, but since you're not down on each of the fours it feels progressively noble, delicate, and sentimental.

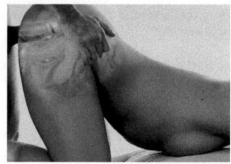

Why it works

- She gets a conceivably orgasmic G-spot rub from his penis as it slides against the front mass of her vagina on each push.
- It claims to her "being taken" dreams since she simply needs to lie still and get him.
- He has simple access and finishes the opportunity of development since he's lying in the middle of her legs; in addition to he gets that sentiment of control.
- The way that you're not eye to eye makes it simple to enjoy a private dream.

You can tailor the situation to your disposition: make it warm and sentimental for delicate cherishing, or fun-loving and unusual for wild evenings in.

Chapter 6 Anal sex

Anal sex is something that not everyone has had experience with. It has the potential to provide you and your partner with very great pleasure if you know how to safely and comfortably engage in this type of sex. In this chapter, I will explain how you can safely have anal sex and how you can begin to use it to your advantage in order to experience pleasure like never before.

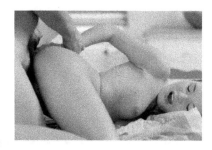

Your First Time

As I mentioned, there are some things to keep in mind when having anal sex for the first number of times. Below, I will outline these points so that you can approach your first anal sex experiences with confidence.

1. Lubrication

The key to anal sex is lubrication! You will need to make sure that both the penis (or dildo) and the anus are well-lubricated in order for anal sex to be pleasurable for everyone involved. The anus doesn't lubricate itself like the vagina does, so you have to make sure you do it yourselves before having anal sex.

2. Relaxation

The next point to keep in mind is relaxation. The anus will open gradually as you start to play around and inside of it a little bit. As you slide something into it, it will respond by opening up and relaxing, but this may take a few minutes. Having the person be relaxed and comfortable is very important. Remember to let it do its thing, and just slowly enjoy the process without rushing it. If the person is too nervous, it will take longer for their anus to relax.

3. Removal

The next thing to note is that if you are going to remove something like a toy or a penis from the anus, it is important to make sure the person is relaxed and lubricated (as stated above). More importantly, they must be expecting the removal of whatever was inserted into their anus to happen. If you try to quickly remove it without the person expecting it, their body will reflexively tense the anus, and it will lead to a painful experience, possibly for both people if it was a penis inserted.

Remembering these three points will help you to have a positive and enjoyable anal sex experience for your first time. There are a few more things to note in order to ensure that you have safe anal sex. These points are related to hygiene and sex toys and will likely become more relevant when you are more experienced with anal sex. As mentioned previously, you are not required to buy two different toys- one for anal and one for vaginal use, but it is important to remember that if something was in your anus or anyone else's, you want to wash it thoroughly before you insert it near or into your vagina or near or into anyone else's vagina. The reason for this is because there are bacteria in the anus that when brought into the vagina or near the urethra can lead to an infection of the bladder. In order to avoid this, after using an anal sex toy or after inserting a penis into the anus with a condom on it, wash the sex toy thoroughly with soap and hot water, or change the condom. If you used a toy anally- say a dildo, and you want to use it vaginally in the same session, make sure to either put a condom on it both times but switch the condom in between, put a condom on it for anal sex and take it off for vaginal sex or use it for anal sex, wash it and then put a condom on it for vaginal sex.

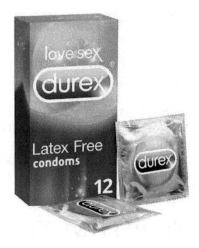

Finally, when using any sort of toys anally, make sure that they are either long enough so that they cannot be inserted all the way in, or if they are not as long as this, (like anal beads or a butt plug), ensure that they have a ring or a handle on the end so that you can easily remove them when you are ready to take them out. If they do not have a ring or a handle or some means of being removed, do not insert them into your anus. This is because it would be easy to get something stuck in your anus. The reason this can happen is that when trying to remove something from the anus with your fingers, the anus will use a reflex that closes the sphincter and will make it very, very difficult to retrieve anything. If you are trying to use your fingers to get it out and the anus closes up on you reflexively, there will not be enough space inside for you to grab onto the toy, and you will just end up pushing it farther into the anus. This will end up causing more of a problem.

Kama Sutra Positions for Anal Sex

The following positions are great for people who are new to anal sex and would like to try some of the simpler positions in order to get used to the feeling of anal sex. These positions are straight from the Kama Sutra, or slight variations of Kama Sutra positions in order to make the optimized for anal sex.

Oral With Anal Stimulation

This first position is not involving anal penetration with a penis but is a great introduction to anal play. This position is done when a woman is giving a man oral sex. The man stands up and the woman is on her knees in front of him, giving him oral sex. She will then reach around behind the man's buttocks and stimulate his anus with her finger. She can move her finger around the outside of his anus, stimulating the sensitive skin there which will make him feel immense amounts of pleasure. Giving oral sex and stimulating his anus at the same time will make it virtually impossible for him not to orgasm very quickly.

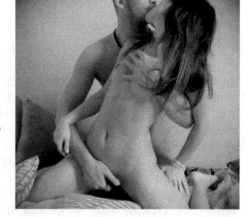

The Curled Angel

This is a Kama Sutra position that is written as a position to be performed with vaginal sex, but it can also be done as an anal sex position. This position involves the man and woman lying down on their sides, the man behind the woman. Both of them are facing the same direction, so the curve of their hips places the man's penis at the perfect point for anal penetration. In this position, the man and woman can grind their hips into each other, and it is a team effort in terms of control.

The Clip

In this position, the man lies back on the bed with his knees bent and his feet planted on the bed. The woman straddles the man and inserts his penis into her anus. In this position, she can lean forward onto the man's bent knees for support, and she is able to control the depth and speed of penetration. The man can hold onto the woman's buttocks and guide her movements as well.

The Snake

This position is a good one to try when you have a little bit of experience with anal sex but are not ready to try anything too extreme just yet. The person receiving anal penetration in this position takes a passive role and can just focus on relaxing and enjoying the pleasure rather than having to contort into some type of acrobatic formation.

To begin, the woman will lie face down on the bed, and her partner will lie on top of her, supporting himself with his arms. From here, the woman will arch her back a bit to make her pleasure zones as accessible as possible for penetration. Now, the man will slowly slide his penis into her anus. Here, the woman can enjoy the pleasure ride her partner takes her on, without having to do anything herself. She is able to enjoy these moments where the focus is all on her!

Pegging

There is another type of anal sex that can be had, which involves sex toys. It is quite common that a woman will penetrate her male partner anally while wearing a strap-on. This practice is called Pegging. Now that you know a little more about sex toys and anal sex, and how to ensure you are combining these two in a safe and sanitary way, you are ready to try Pegging. This can be done either by using a dildo placed in a strap-on that a woman is wearing or by using a double-ended dildo. Using a double-ended dildo will allow the woman to be pleasured at the same time as she is penetrating the man, as she will also be penetrated either vaginally or anally with the other end of the dildo. This type of dildo looks like any other, except that it has two identical ends.

Now that you are aware of the possibility of this type of practice, you can understand how any of these anal sex positions can be performed by either the man penetrating the woman anally with his penis or by the woman penetrating her partner anally using a dildo.

For men, anal sex is extremely pleasurable since their prostate is stimulated through anal penetration. The prostate is what has been referred to as the "male G-Spot."

These moves are a collection of beginner, intermediate and pro anal positions. They allow for varying amounts of penetration and stimulation. If you are brand new to anal, we suggest trying one that has both partners side by side, or the lady on top so she can control the movements and speed. If you are more experienced, feel free to try any of these.

The Curled Angel

This sex move is a variation of the sexy spoons position. It allows for intimate closeness, and gives both parties the ability to control the speed and depth of penetration. It works by having the lady laying on whichever side is most comfortable for her. She should have her knees pulled up towards her chest, exposing her bottom to him. The gentleman can then slide in behind her, holding her with his arms, and tuck his legs up under hers. From there, he can penetrate her, and they can work together to control the penetration and intimacy involved in this position.

Double Decker

This is a woman on top position that actually gives the man a little more control, but keeps the majority of it with the woman. It is a wonderful position for those who are a little more experienced with anal, or who are good with balance, as slipping could lead to a potentially painful accident. To do it, have the gentleman lay on his back on the bed. He can have his legs outstretched in whatever position is comfortable for him. The lady can then lay on her back over top of him, then prop herself up with her elbows and feet. From there, he can help guide her on to his penis and control the penetration, while she controls the speed and depth at which he enters.

Rocking Horse

This is an intimate woman on top position that allows both lovers to engage in a sensual make out session at the same time. It works by having the gentleman sitting up, then leaning back on his hands. His knees can either be bent up to create a seat for her, or his legs can be stretched out to give her free space. Then, the lady can straddle over top of him with a leg on either side of his waist, and guide his penis to penetrate her from behind. From there, she can proceed to control the depth, speed and rhythm, while both lovers enjoy a deep and loving gaze, or a sexy make out session.

Reverse Cowgirl

A book of sex moves just isn't complete without the reverse cowgirl. As luck would have it, this position is a wonderful opportunity for a woman on top anal move. To engage in this position, start by having him lay on his back in whatever way is comfortable for him. Then, she can straddle him with her back towards his face. She can continue to control the depth and speed of penetration, while giving him a sexy view of her bum as it bounces up and down on him.

Doggy Style

The classic doggy style happens to be one of the best positions for anal penetration. It allows the gentleman to have almost full control over thrusting, so he should take care to ensure he is not being too vigorous for her, and she should take care to communicate how it feels for her. To do this position, the lady should get on all fours. Then, the gentleman can sit on his knees behind her, and enter her slowly, working up to a steady rhythm until he cums.

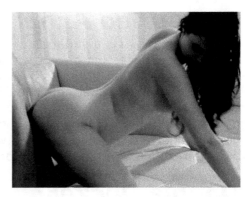

Glowing Triangle

This intimate face to face position is one of the best for anal sex. It is a man on top position that allows for deep penetration, but due to the angle it can inadvertently cause g-spot stimulation at the same time. Ideally, you should have a pillow involved to make this a more comfortable position. To get into form, start by having the lady lay on her back with the cushion under the small of her back holding her bum up in the air. Her knees should be bent with her feet firmly on the bed, helping hold her up and exposed. The gentleman can then slide in between her legs and penetrate her, while she hugs him. For added stimulation, she can use a free hand to rub her clitoris. This is a very sensual position for anal sex that is excellent for a romantic anal experience.

Reclining Lotus

This is basically an expansion of the Glowing Triangle, but allows for even more g-spot stimulation through deep penetration. It starts by having the lady laying on her back. Using a pillow under the small of her back helps her expose her anus to the gentleman, so it is ideal to have one handy for this position. Then, she should bend her knees up towards her chest, while letting her legs spread out sideways. The gentleman can then slide up in between her legs and penetrate her bum while keeping his face close to hers. She can either hook her feet under his thighs, or lock her legs behind his back. It is a wonderful position for nuzzling each other or having a steamy make out session while having sex.

Afternoon Delight

This is a fun variation of a spooning position that allows for deep penetration while giving the man the majority of the control. It is a very relaxed position that allows you to lovingly gaze into each other's eyes, or simply enjoy the moment. It starts by having the gentleman laying on whatever side is more comfortable for him, with his knees slightly bent for balance. Then, the lady lays on her back on a 90-degree angle from him, with her bum lined up to his penis. He can then penetrate her and thrust at whatever speed and depth is comfortable for the both of them.

The Amazon

This is a lady on top position that requires a chair or a stool to be done. It can be a very sensual move that allows for nuzzling and romancing while engaging in some delightful anal sex. To start, the gentleman should sit comfortably on a seat that has no arms. Then, the lady can mount him, while facing him, and having a leg on either side. She can continue to control the thrusting for whatever is most comfortable for her. Either the gentleman or the lady can use a spare hand to stimulate her clitoris or breasts (or both!) to add to the pleasure of this move.

The Basket

This position is a lady on top move that allows for both parties to have almost equal control over the movements. The basket allows for both lovers to face one another, and have a free hand for additional stimulation to enhance the move. To start, the gentleman should sit on a comfortable surface with his legs out straight. He should be sitting up enough that he doesn't have to use his hands to support himself. Then, the lady can straddle him with a leg on either side of his waist, while controlling the penetration. She can use his shoulders for leverage, while he puts his hands under her bum to help lift her up and down on his penis. This move allows for you to move as slowly or as quickly as you desire.

Chapter 7 Pre-love Game. Secrets

Unique Prelude

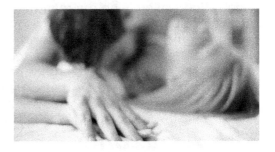

The concept of foreplay is pervasive. It includes and getting to know each other, and the time of the mutual sexual interest, and the so-called foreplay (kissing, mutual nudity, fondling, erotic massages), and much more.

Before you make contact, you must reliably ensure that your desire is mutual. Many partners do not burden themselves with the conventions and talk about their desire to have sex openly. But many people have this shy or afraid of being rejected. However, many thousands of people have come up with a massive number of ways to communicate their sexual desire without any words. Looks, smiles, and gestures are often able to convey much more than words helpless and insecure.

If you intend to show your beloved or chosen one that he or she is causing your sexual interest, try to delay his gaze a little longer than is usually accepted. In ordinary conversation, face to face or in the company attempts to reduce the physical distance between himself and the object of your desire, provoke "casual," "accidentally" touch. Sit so that your knees feel each other, casually touch his arm or chest. Just try to make it as natural as possible and relaxed, without pressure, pressure and open manifestations of "Basic Instinct," otherwise you will likely scare away your potential partner.

If you find that your partner responds positively to your "accidentally" touch, then it's time to move on to something more — for example, a kiss.

Kiss - one of the most common types of lovemaking. Kiss capable of expressing a variety of emotions - from soft and friendly to the care-consuming erotic arousal and desire. Ancient Taoist writings, for example, emphasize the importance of deep sensory kissing, placing them in second place directly after intercourse. And, in fact, can give kiss lovers with nothing incomparable feeling of genuine intimacy with each other.

In the East, the kisses have always been a profoundly intimate part of lovemaking. Until now, almost impossible to see the Indian or Chinese couples who kiss in the open on the street. The same applies to the movie: until recently, the scene of the kiss could not be seen in any of the east films.

Most of the different cultures recognize kiss ideal for a whole range of expressions of human emotions - from a friendly welcome to the erotic energy exchange. However, in many African, Polynesian, and other tribes living in primitive society, a kiss is virtually unknown. So, for example, Eskimos greet and caress each different rubbing noses, while focusing on the mutual exchange of breath and a slight, subtle smell of leather.

Ancient Indian love treatises recognize the importance of a kiss. The most famous esoteric teachings of Eastern Tantra calls Kiss to contact the Upper Gate. When the couple is passionately kissing, says Kama Sutra, the partners are crumbling all barriers and boundaries. The kiss symbolizes the state of maximum readiness of both parties for rapprochement and unification of the lingam and yoni. The Indian treatises are stating that the shape and size of the female yoni can be identified by the shape and size of the female's mouth. The size of the lingam is determined by the length of the nose man. You, too, have heard about it? Therefore, this wisdom for thousands of years handed down from generation to generation and was known to the ancient Indians for many centuries before the Christian era.

Erotic kissing provides an excellent opportunity to explore both male and female qualities. Partners often change roles, as their tongues penetrate each other's mouths. Thus, a kiss can be successfully used to study the movements and rhythms that can later be transferred to the motion Lingam and Yonis.

Kama Sutra indicates the following places and body parts that are most appropriate for kissing: the forehead, eyes, cheeks, lips, neck, chest and arms, thighs, stomach, and yoni. Kissing in compliance with a specific sequence of points in the body helps to awaken all the richness and diversity of the senses.

The most common opinion is that women kiss much more critical than for men, although it is men who initiated the kissing act much more frequently. To excite a woman kissing, you must know what she likes. Some women prefer a lighter touch surface; other strokes stimulate the lips or tongue inner surface of the lips. Others are excited by the fact that the partner sucks them the upper or lower lip. The most exciting is considered to be a kiss, in which both partners to penetrate the language in the mouth of each other and make them stroking or Jog.

Kama Sutra lists the three types of kisses that are most suitable for young women. The first is called a superficial kiss; with this kiss, lips, lovers barely touching. The second type - a tremulous kiss; in this case, the woman moves her lower lip, while the man presses his lips to her mouth. The third type - the real kiss, and here she uses the language.

> **Also in the Kama Sutra describes other types of kisses.**
>
> - In direct kiss, lovers are in direct contact with lips.
> - Trailing kiss, both partners are attracted to each other heads.
> - When raised, one partner kisses another raising his head, holding it by the chin.
> - When kissing, a lip is pressed toward the partner firmly.
> - In pressed great kiss, his lower lip held concerning the language and firmly pressed against her.
> - In a final kiss, one partner completely covers the lips of another.

When the Battle of languages is one of the partners comes to his tongue and palate another language.

There is another classification of Kama Sutra kisses, which seemed to be the most user-friendly, poetic, sensual, and more. Having mastered all of these options, the lovers will be able to enrich and diversify your sexual arsenal significantly.

1. **Bashfully** - woman showering lips partners with short, frequent, small kisses, moving in such a way as if trying to break away from him.
2. **A playful** - woman is moving the tongue in the mouth of the partner, and at this time, he gently bites her lips.
3. **Flat** - man must bind his lips partner's lips and draw them, trying to touch her tongue.
4. **Exquisite** - Partners stroke languages palate each other.
5. **Inati** - partners must caressing each lip portion to each other, not touching the teeth.
6. **Ata** - a man and a woman, should try to push your tongue a language partner.
7. **The most** - the man must embrace the female lips tongue and suck it, just nipping teeth.
8. **Tenderness** - partners lip gently stroking each other's language.
9. **Sari** - the man, gently kisses the palm of a woman, as well as the inner surfaces of the hands, lips moving from the bottom up, from wrist to armpit.
10. **Mill** - the man, rotates the woman tongue with his tongue, pressing it to her cheeks and the palate.
11. **Petala** - the man should put his tongue in her cheek and rotate it.
12. **Kiss teeth** - a man, his head thrown back a woman, his tongue across her lips, and she bites his tongue.
13. **Sink** - a kiss on the ear with a slight sucking and biting the ear lobe.
14. **Duel mouths** - partners must draw each other's lips, slightly biting them.

Men should also be aware of the fact that one of the most sensitive areas on the body of a woman is the external border of the lips. And therefore, we should not forget the gentle stroking movements of the tongue around his lips partner.

Particular attention Tantric treatises give the so-called secret of the upper lip. The upper lip is a woman - not just another erogenous zone of the female body. It is particularly sensitive, according to the Tantra teachers, because of the palate and upper lip of a woman connected to her clit through the thin nerve canal. Tantric writings refer to this Nerve Canal This Snail Wisdom, as it is believed that he was in his tender parts spiraling like a shell. Tantrikas claim that the kiss of the upper lip, as well as oral sex with clitoral stimulation, creates a unique energy circulation within the female body. Massage the upper lip releases sexual energy and stimulates sexual desire.

And Kama Sutra and Ananga-ranga describe kisses with the upper lip. A man can excite the top rim of a woman, gently biting and sucking on it, while a woman is playing with his lower lip with the help of the teeth and tongue. If both use the teeth so as not to cause pain, but create a wave of pleasure, then this practice may be fascinating for both partners.

Tantrikas believe that a woman can visualize the channel connecting her clitoris with the upper lip. Presenting it in your mind as a hollow vibrating tube, the bottom of which is twisted into a helix, a woman may consciously spend on its sexual energy flows. Stimulate this channel you can use the deep breathing combined with muscle contractions of the vagina. By learning to control this secret nerve duct, a woman will be able to increase the pleasure of love for yourself and your partner.

From kissing caressing move to hand movements. Some men often do not know what to do with your hands during a love game. The solution is elementary - hand man must be in constant motion. You can alternately stroke their thighs, buttocks, and breasts partner, massage your shoulder blades and neck, to hold down the top of the neck, back, touching the tips of his fingers abdomen. Almost all women strongly excited when they caress nipples. Nipple stimulation can produce a man with his fingertips, stroking them, squeezing or pinching.

Partners must deliver great fun from the process of mutual undressing. It is essential not to hurry and not to throw all my clothes immediately. Provide partner gradually discover your body esteem and feel the difference between the touch of the body parts in clothing and bare skin. Also, many men experience sexual arousal on the type of clothes, and they like to make love with a partially dressed woman. You cannot remove the bra and lace stockings. You can also stay in a semi-transparent combination, thereby unlocking the imagination of a man and letting him get all that is hidden under clothing.

Many men get turned black lingerie color, others like apricot or golden flesh, the same or similar in hue to the partner's body. Lace underwear red stimulates excess production of sex hormones in men and from ancient times the color associated with sensual pleasure. In Eastern cultures, red and white have mystical and symbolic properties. The white color associated with the male principle and the red was a symbol of women, sexuality, creative force, and a successful, happy life. In ancient China, the bride wore red silk trousers, and the wedding was called Red betrothal.

In Islamic tradition, the red color attributed similar qualities, Muslims use the word "red" in the sense of "beautiful," referring to a beautiful woman Red maid. The red veil is considered particularly seductive. "If you go out, my girl, put on the red veil," - advised a famous Arab poet.

The red color in the Tantric tradition symbolizes fire. Red Dakini, the Tantric Goddess of ecstasy, looks like a young girl, full of passion, and signifies the freshness of feelings. In India and Tibet, men and women painted on the forehead small red circles, seeing them as a sign of identification with Kundalini - inner creative energy.

During foreplay, women should not ignore the body of the partner. In addition to the genital area of men have sexual sensitivity, and other areas of the body. But many women, clearly knowing that the stimulation of the penis leads him into a state of alert, often do not even think about what could bring a partner to the limit of excitement, caressing the tongue and lips, for example, the fingers of his hands or feet. Each man has his own hidden erogenous hiding place, the existence of which often does not know himself.

Both partners strongly excited by accidental contact with the genitals. During lovemaking, the woman can hold abreast of the member of the partner. You may also cling to the outer surface of the genitals of the thigh.

The action of warm water can not only remove excess voltage but also prepare the body for a more sensitive and heightened perception of touches and strokes. Take a hot bath, apply a body lotion or cream flavored, and then easily touch the skin favorite in the most secluded corners of the body. Repeat here that you love him endlessly and feel very sexy. At the same time, let him know that you are very much excited about his affection and ask him to repeat them again and again. Do not be afraid to talk about their feelings, sincerely and naturally.

Men need to remember that the water washes away the natural lubrication of a woman, and therefore of the stimulation of the clitoris and vagina in water is better to abstain.

Oriental treatises on the art of love always contain sections on the bites and scratches: bites and scrapes partner - the perfect way to express strong feelings. Teeth and nails can be used deliberately to stimulate the erogenous zones. Smooth biting earlobes, gentle biting the neck - like Tiger does this with a tigress - very exciting. Hill Venus in the female genitalia and the base of the spine are also those zones playful biting, which gives a pleasant feeling.

The most common a love bite, known in the West - is sucked or tingling of the skin of the partner. As a result of the taste (Suction) on the body is a red speck, like a small bruise. Such love bruises - a powerful reminder of the recent experiences the bliss of love, they remain a long time, and many men are proud to show them around.

The Kama Sutra says: "Lovers can bite the same place that you can kiss, except for sensitive areas such as the upper lip, mouth, and eyes."

Kama Sutra lists seven different types of love bites, which are classified following what marks after them remain on the skin lovers.

- Secret sting when the skin is reddened.
- Swollen bite, when the bite swells.
- Spot bite when the marks are only from two teeth on the small area of skin.
- When a small area of skin has prints of all teeth.
- Coral Jewelry, and when used at the same time, kissing and teeth, and lips, while the lips are called coral, and the teeth - precious stones.
- Broken Cloud when chest bite mouth wide open.
- Bite Boar - most passionate, furious, animal kiss, wherein lovers lose control. After this, a kiss is still a lot of full rows, which are located not far from each other, the marks on the shoulders or chest, skin intervals between which the red.

Next, Kama Sutra points to some regions of the body, where it is best to make certain types of bites. Deep bite, as well as puffiness and spot bites, is best done on the lower lip of the partner: throats, armpits, and outer thighs.

The Kama Sutra states that bites can be incorporated into foreplay only if the woman is nice. A woman should bite her partner back with a vengeance - and this inflames it.

"When a man bites a woman, she should do the same thing with a vengeance. Thus, the bite point must be returned in the form of the Rosary, and in retribution for making rosary woman Broken Cloud. If a woman feels that she teased, it has to "fight" with a partner, and immediately. In this case, it must grab her lover by the hair, bend his head down to kiss him on his upper lip, and then close your eyes and bite him in various places ", - stated in the Kama Sutra.

If love bites gently, skillfully, and delicately woven into the pre-game, then it leads to mutual sensual pleasure partners.

In ancient India, the nails often specially prepared to ensure that they use them while making love matches. "Especially passionate lovers must obtain nails of his left hand so that they looked like a miniature chain saw with two or three teeth," - says the Kama Sutra.

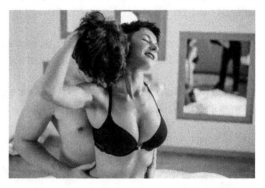

On the Eastern erotic paintings often depicted traces of polish on the naked bodies of the lovers. Picturesque, this technique has been used by artists to demonstrate: Lovers achieved complete satisfaction. Indeed, quite often covered by passion and desire intoxicated, lovers dig her nails into the skin of the partner quite unconsciously, without thinking about it.

"Lover, with tenderness and passion touching his beloved, can bring great comfort to her. There is nothing more than delivering excitement and fun wife and husband than the skillful use of nails." - says another ancient Indian treatise of love, Ananga-ranga.

Eight different types of nail markings are described in Kama Sutra Ananga-ranga.

- **Sounding** - pressing, after which almost no trace.
- **Crescent** - the trace of a nail.
- **Circle** - two crescents that face each other. Such nip trace remains after two nails.

- **Line of passion** - a long straight mark that remains after spending the nail on the skin.
- **Claw of the Tiger** - a curve, score, similar to the one that leaves the claw of beast.
- **Peacock** - an imprint of all five nails.
- **Jump hare** - a track on which all five marks of the pins are very close to each other.
- **Blue lotus leaf** - mark resembling a sheet and its shape made nails of one hand.

According to Oriental authors, through the energy of nails can be carried out - to transmit its internal power to your partner. Long nails can cause in your lover or with the incomparable pleasure. That's what says about this Ananga-rank "Lover connecting tenderness and passion in their touch to the beloved, can bring great comfort to her. There are nothing more delivering excitement and fun for wife and husband than the skilful use of nails. "

Embrace - This is another important element of foreplay. In a broad sense, any contact between lovers - this is some form of arms. Embrace accompany the whole act of love - from foreplay to passionate intertwining of the limbs at the approach of mutual ecstasy. Even when the lovers take each other's hand, weaving his fingers, it is also considered a "hug fingers." The expression of love is carried out primarily employing arms. The Kama Sutra states that shampooing your partner - also a form of weapons.

Kama Sutra and the Anangu-grade describes eight types of hugs.

Wrapping, like ivy: Both partners are. A woman hugs her partner as plastic ivy twines around a tree trunk. Lifting his foot, she throws her on the thigh lover repeatedly kisses him and pulls his head to her.

Climbing a tree: A man stands firm, the woman puts one of his foot on his foot, and the other raises the level of the hips partner and eagerly pressed him. She wraps both hands around his waist as if trying to climb a palm tree. She pressed against the "tree trunk" with all possible force. Twisting, it kisses it as avidly as if drinking the water of life.

A mixture of rice and sesame seeds: It can be practiced to embrace both standing and lying down. Partners in this type of hugs should hold each other so tightly to the thigh, and one hand was thoroughly pressed against the legs and arms of another. Between the two wings and thighs is mutual friction. At this point, the partner can touch the lingam yoni, and for some time to remain pressed against her.

The mixture of milk and water: Partners passionately embrace each other as if seeking to penetrate the body of a loved one. Their arms and legs entwined. This embrace of standing can be performed while sitting and lying.

The embrace of the breasts: A man should squeeze her nipples to the breast's partner. He must sit very close, almost close to it, and thus should keep their eyes closed.

Embrace of foreheads: When lovers are in contact and pressed against each other heads, which means that they show great trepidation and great tenderness. They may then hug each other around the waist, so that not only their foreheads but the lips, breasts, bellies touched.

Embrace the middle part: The man firmly presses the hips and thighs of women to their own. This type of hug delivers the greatest pleasure in sitting position, regardless of whether the woman is sitting on your partner or vice versa.

Embrace the thighs: One of the lovers must with force to compress one or both hips partner her hips. This type of hug can be practiced in a variety of poses.

Of course, these eight types referred to above do not exhaust all the options embrace. Kama Sutra says in this regard that during the next permissible and even necessary to practice all possible hugs, including those that are not described in the special love treatises. None of the hugs are prohibited if it does not cause pain to your partner and inflames his passion. "When the Wheel of Love is set in motion - says Kama Sutra - there is no longer any clear rules." This means that the lover is intended for the most extensive field of improvisation, for the realization of the most bizarre of their desires and fantasies. Embrace - the best way to establish harmony in the emotions of women and men. Love hugs used as a preparation for copulation, help partners overcome all differences, a sense of alienation, lack of mutual understanding.

All the cares of the world, all the fears, all the mutual distrust are dissolved in a passionate embrace of souls and bodies. "No matter what thought for a moment the man, for whatever care a woman, no matter what may have been imagined in their heads, they disappear entirely. And nothing else exists in this world - a man and a woman in embrace fused."

Chapter 8 Positions Of Kamasutra

Bandoleer
While the woman lays on her back and lifts the two knees up towards her chest, the man stoops facing her. She can then lay her feet on his chest while he places his forearms on her knees. The woman can then grab the man's thighs and draw him closer to more profound penetration. The more he pushes down on her knees, the greater the pleasure for her.

A relatively straightforward sex position, which doesn't require too much flexibility.

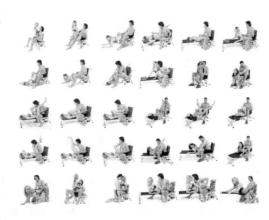

Widely Open
The Widely Open requires a touch of male chest area solidarity to hold for any time allotment. The female lies on the bed; a pad is propped under her head. She lifts her knees toward her chest, marginally lifting her bottom off the bed. Her partner is one of his knees when he approaches her. He slides between her legs, plunks down without anyone else ankles, and penetrates from this seated position. The chest area quality comes in as he places his hands under her back, lifting her body up and toward him in a thrusting movement.

Dolphin
The Dolphin requires a ton of versatility and quality. The female accomplice lies on the floor, squeezing her feet down as she raises her back and bottoms off the ground. The male accomplice gently opens her legs and slides between her thighs for entrance. The propelled Dolphin includes the male accomplice setting his hands under the base of his accomplice and lifting up until her feet leave the floor. The weight on the neck of the female accomplice can be extreme, so don't hold the situation for a really long time.

Twofold Decker
Double Decker is a transitional sex position perfect for moving, beginning with one position then onto the following. The male deceptions face-up on his back. The female plunks down on the male with her back to him, permitting

infiltration. She at that point reclines, putting her elbows on the bed. Her elbows hold her body weight. The female at that point bends her knees and spots her feet on the knees of her male accomplice. The male controls beat and entrance. To progress to another position, the male just rolls the female.

Falcon or Eagle

The Eagle is one of the less mind boggling sex position. The female lies back and lifts her legs with her feet highlighted the roof. She at that point spreads her legs as far separated as agreeable. Her accomplice stoops with knees spread for entrance. The male accomplice can grasp her legs for help, to direct rhythm or enter further. She can essentially lay back or give a little consideration to herself.

Fan

The Fan is a fundamental sexual position that takes into account significant entrance. The male and female stand upstanding, her back is confronting his front. She bends around a little table or seat and lays her weight on her lower arms. He comes in from the other side, takes hold of her hips, and infiltrates. The male controls all advancement, infiltration significance, speed, and musicality. This position likewise works with the female twisting around the bed.

Fabulous Rocking Horse style

The Fantastic Rocking Horse is a position by which female-on-top position best performed on a hard surface like the floor. The male accomplice sits on the floor leg over the leg. He should recline on his arms to help his weight or incline toward a divider or other hard article to free his hands. The female accomplice straddles her accomplice, embracing his thighs with her thighs. The female controls infiltration and speed. The Fantastic Rocking Horse requires thigh quality. If the female accomplice gets worn out, the male accomplice can use his free hands to assist quiet with weighting on thigh muscles by snatching the sides of her base and helping control infiltration.

Overlay or fold

If the male accomplice is normally versatile, the Fold might be an incredible situation to endeavor. The female lies on her back, ideally on the floor. She bends her knees insignificantly and spreads her legs wide. The male plunks down on the bed, the legs outstretched. He slides his legs on either side of her body while pulling his body between her thighs. She should lift her feet off the ground immediately as he positions himself in the right spot. She lifts her base to permit entrance as he curves forward, folding his arms over her midsection during infiltration.

Frog

The Frog is a situated sexual position that uses the edge of the bed for fitting situating. The male will sit on the cornered edge of the bed with one leg on each side of the corner. The female hunches down before her accomplice, back confronting him. He directs entrance from behind. Be that as it may, she controls beat and significance of infiltration. The male can put his hands on his accomplice's hips to help decrease the strain on her muscles.

G-Force

The G-Force is a fun sex position that requires a touch of adaptability on the female's part. The female lies on her back, pulling her knees in carefully shrouded. Her male partner approaches from behind, grabbing hold of her feet/legs and lifting her bottom off the floor. Her weight is moved to her upper shoulders and neck as her bottom is positioned near her partner's penis.
He entered from this position and control development and beat. For added pleasure, she can place her feet on his chest, allowing him to grab her hips for more profound penetration.

Galley

The Galley is a sexual position achieved with the male sitting on the bed or other hard surface. His legs ought to be loosened up straight. The female straddles his hips, her bottom facing his chest. Her weight is supported on her upper arms. She slides her bottom back and down, allowing the penis to penetrate. She controls development, cadence, and profundity. His hands are completely allowed to massage and explore her body.

Glowing Juniper

The Glowing Juniper is a romantic sexual position. The female rests on the bed, legs outstretched, and somewhat spread. The male slides into position between her legs, leaving his legs outstretched as well. He wraps his hands around her waist and lifts marginally to position her body for penetration. On the off chance that he's adaptable enough, he can lean over and kiss her tummy in this position or basically clutch her body and investigate her eyes.

Glowing Triangle

The Glowing Triangle resembles the classic Missionary, yet there is a wind. The female lays on her back with legs far enough apart for her partner to settle near her body. He places his knees down on the bed and his hands on either side of his partner's head. The female partner then lifts her hips by pushing up with her feet, controlling penetration and speed. A wedge can be utilized under her bottom or lower back to lessen the strain on the legs and back.

Grasp

The Grip is straightforward, however profoundly powerful — the female lies on her back with a pad placed under her hips for a little stature. Her legs are apart sufficiently far to allow her penetration, the female lifts her legs, wrap them around her partner and places her feet on his bottom. She has taken control of the position, moving her hips and pelvis to pleasure her partner.

Hero

The Hero is a sexual position that gives the female partner a touch of time to rest. The female lies flat on the bed. She pulls her knees toward her chest, stretching her feet to the ceiling. Her bottom is marginally raised off the bed as her male partner slides his knees under her bottom for penetration. The male partner can push down on the back of the thighs, pushing them toward her belly to change the vaginal angle for better penetration.

Hinge

The Hinge is a position similar to the Doggy Style. The female in on all fours; however, her weight is on her forearms rather than her hands. Her legs are spread apart side. Her partner approaches from behind on his knees. One knee slides between her legs, and the other is outstretched. She is in charge of development with the Hinge. She pushes ahead and backward, shifting her weight to shake the position after penetration.

Indrani

The Indrani is ideal for men who are plentifully supplied. The female lies back on the bed with a pad propping up her head. She lifts her knees and destroys them into her chest. Her feet are spread marginally apart. He approaches her bottom on his knees. With her bottom in the air, he can penetrate from behind. Her legs are on either side of his chest, under his arms, and his arms are by his knees. He is leaning forward, moving his hips to push.

Stoop/kneel

The Kneel is best performed on the floor or another hard surface. The male and female partner faces each other, both on their knees (however not hands and knees). His thighs are pressed together so she can straddle him for penetration. She can clutch his neck for support, and he can wrap his arms around her waist to pull her nearby and support a portion of her weight. The face to face position is ideal for kissing.

Landslide

The Landslide is a marginally troublesome position to achieve, yet it gives a more tightly fit upon penetration. The female lies on her stomach with her chest area weight positioned on her forearms. Her legs are loosened up straight, marginally parted. The male sits just underneath her bottom at her thighs. He leans back, supporting his weight on his arms extended behind him. He penetrates from this position. After penetration, she shuts her legs for a more tightly fit.

Lotus Blossom

In the Lotus Blossom, both the male and female partners sit leg over leg. This position requires the two partners to be marginally adaptable. The male sits on the floor in the lotus (with folded legs) position. His female partner approaches from the front, sitting on his lap for penetration. Her legs wrap around his body. She can utilize her bottom, legs, and arms to climb, down, left, and right from the Lotus Blossom position. His hands can slide under her bottom or grasp her hips to aid development.

Prurient Leg

The female partner must be very adaptable to achieve the Lustful Leg position. The two partners stand facing each other. The female lifts her advantage toward the ceiling, resting her all-inclusive leg on her partners shoulder. She is essentially performing a standing split. Penetration can happen before or after she raises her leg. The male can place his hands on her hips for leverage and more profound penetration.

Magic Mountain

This fun sexual position requires building a mountain of pads first. Stack three to four cushions on top of each other, leaving enough room behind the pads for the two partners to lean over the stack. The female partner leans over the pads. First, thighs pressed together. The male partner approaches from behind, snuggling up near the female. He places his knees on the outside of her legs using his feet to guide penetration and cadence.

Mermaid

The Mermaid is an interesting position that can be achieved with the female partner lying on the floor or a waist-high table. The female rests on her back, lifting her legs in the air with feet pointed toward the ceiling. The male approaches the female, grabbing on to her lifted legs while he penetrates. He can utilize her legs as a means of leverage or allow them to hang free. Add a bend to the Mermaid by allowing the female partner's legs to fall open widely after penetration.

Nirvana

The Nirvana is a derivation of the classic Missionary. The female partner lays flat on her back with her legs together. She ought to clutch the bedposts or mattresses for leverage. Her partner straddles her legs with his knees, penetrating from the front. Intercourse requires partnered developments with the two partners moving at the same time. The weight of her thighs increases the intensity and allows for clitoral stimulation. On the off chance that penetration is troublesome, she can marginally open her legs, allowing her partner to penetrate the vagina before closing her legs tight again.

Padlock

The Padlock is similar to the Erotic V. The female partner sits on a table or other elevated hard surface. The male partner approaches his partner from the front. He pulls her delicately toward him, so her bottom is marginally off the table. She then leans back, allowing penetration. After penetration, she bolts her legs around his bottom. Depending on the length of the female partner's legs, she may have to lay one leg on each of her partner's bottom cheeks rather than lock her feet around him.

Peg

The Peg is a rather complicated position that may take a little practice to master. The male lies on his side, legs outstretched. The female also rests. However, her head is near his feet. She pulls his thighs between her thighs and embraces on his lower legs with her arms. Her bottom ought to be positioned near his penis. The male can enter from this position and control development and mood.

Furrow /Plough

The Plow requires a great deal of chest area quality with respect to the male partner and trust with respect to the female partner — the female twists around the edge of the bed, resting on her arms. Her legs are on the floor spread far enough apart to allow her male partner to cuddle his body beside hers. The male then lifts the female's legs by the hips and holds the lower half of her body in the air while penetrating.

Inclined Tiger /Prone Tiger

The Prone Tiger is a fun sexual position to attempt. The male sits on the bed or other hard surface, legs outstretched. It is best for the male to sit toward the edge of the bed. The female partner straddles his body, her back to his front. She brings down herself onto his penis from the straddling position. After penetration, she extends her legs as straight as conceivable. The female partner grabs on her partner's feet for leverage.

Propeller

In case you're feeling a little adventurous, you can attempt the Propeller. The female lies back on the bed, her legs loosened up and thighs somewhat apart. The male lays his body on top of the female, straddling her midriff, feet toward her head. From this position, he should guide the penis into the vagina for penetration. Penetrating at this angle can be troublesome, so a few men favor entering from a kneeling position and lying down after penetrating.

Proposal

The Proposal is a kneeling sexual position that takes a touch of practice — both the male and female bow down on the floor. The bed may be too soft for this position. Partners are facing each other in the kneeling position. He's on one knee – as if proposing marriage. She mirrors his position and tenderly pushes ahead, placing her deserted foot his left (kneeling) leg. He may have to squat down somewhat for penetration; however, once penetration is achieved, partners can shake back and forth gradually to appreciate the action.

Reclining Lotus

The Reclining Lotus requires the female to have the option to sit in the lotus yoga position. The lotus position is the same as sitting with folded legs. Once in the position, the female lays back on the bed, she crossed legs in the air. The male supports his weight on his arms as he penetrates from the top. Placing a pad under her bottom changes the angle of the vagina and penetration. The cushion also assists ease with pressuring placed on her body if his arms grow somewhat drained.

Switch Cowgirl

The Reverse Cowgirl is one of the more popular sexual positions. The male lies back on the bed, legs outstretched. The female straddles his legs with her bottom facing his chest area. She brings down onto his penis, allowing penetration before moving down to her knees. From here, she can lean forward, press her hands to his legs and weave here and there as tenderly or frantically as she desires. The male partner can clutch her hips for added support and more profound penetration.

Right Angle

Have a spare cushion in the dining room, kitchen, or living room? The Right Angle is a tabletop position with her comfort in mind. She lies on the table with her head on a pad, and her knees pulled somewhat up toward her chest. He approaches the table and grabs onto her legs and spreads them marginally to cuddle close for penetration. She can slide back on the table marginally to place her feet down to hold her feet in the air. His hands are allowed to roam, grab her breasts, or hang on for a wild ride.

Rock n' Roller

The female lies on her back with a pad under her head for the Rock n' Roller. She lifts her legs pulling her feet toward the wall behind her head. Her body resembles she's about to do a back roll. Her male partner penetrates while on his knees. He can place his hands under her bottom to lift her higher, changing the penetration angle and sensation. A pad can also be utilized to appropriate up her hips to diminish strain.

Rowing Boat

The Rowing Boat is a sitting position that allows the male and female to face each other. The man rests on the bed while the female straddles his legs and brings down onto his penis. He then pushes up to a seated position with lifted knees. She slides down somewhat into a seated position, mirroring her partner. From this position, he can slip his hands under her knees to access to her breasts or under her bottom to guide penetration.

Thigh Master

This woman-on-top position is a fun take on an old favorite – the Reverse Cowgirl. The male lies on his back, yet instead of his legs being loosened up, they are bent at the knee. The female straddles her partner with her back, facing him. She brings down onto his penis and places her knees on the bed. Her correct knee is on the outside of his correct thigh, and her left knee is placed between his legs on the bed. From here, she controls development, using his leg or knee for leverage. In the event that tallness is an issue and she has inconvenience moving here and there while straddling, he can place his hands under her bottom to give her a little lift.

Toad

The Toad may not sound like an affectionate name. However, this sexual position is all about closeness. The female lies on the bed with her knees pulled in toward her chest and spread far apart. Her body looks like a toad in a seated position. Her partner rests on top of her, placing his arms around her neck, pulling her nearby. He enters from the front while she places her feet on the back of his legs just underneath his bottom.

Tominagi

Many of the sexual positions in the Kamasutra are derivations in a basic position. That is the case with the Tominagi. The female lies on her back; her head propped up on a cushion. She pulls her knees in toward her chest. Her partner approaches her on his knees, places her feet on his chest, and grabs her knees for leverage while penetrating. He can lift her legs marginally to change the angle of penetration.

Triumph Arch

The Triumph Arch is a position that ought to be tenderly attempted the first run through around. The male lies face up on the bed. The female straddles her partner in a kneeling position allowing penetration. The male then sits up and places his hands behind his partner's back. He holds tight to his partner's weight while she lies back on his legs, placing her head on the bed between his feet. It may be ideal for extending a long time before attempting this position.

Seated Ball

Adaptability is an unquestionable requirement for the Seated Ball. The male sits on the bed or another hard surface. The female sits on his lap with her back to his chest. Penetration happens from this position. The male lifts his knees somewhat, grabs on to his partner's midriff, and twists over as he pulls her in toward him. The Seated Ball resembles a seated, twisted, spooning position. To make the position more comfortable for her, she can lean forward and grab on to her partner's feet or legs for leverage and support.

Temptation /Seduction

The Seduction requires an adaptable female partner. The female lies back on the bed, her feet tucked under her bottom. She places her hands above her head. The male approaches the female from the top with his legs loosened up straight. He holds his body weight on his forearms, which are placed on the bed. A few females find leaving one leg tucked under her bottom, and the other loosened up straight more comfortable.

Shoulder Stand

In yoga class, there is an advanced move called the Shoulder Stand. The sexual position definitely looks like a yoga position — the female lies on her back on the bed. A harder surface like the floor may be more appropriate. She places her arms on the floor and presses up while lifting her legs toward the ceiling. He approaches her on his knees, grabs her bottom, and enters from behind. Her weight ought to be fixated on her upper shoulders, accordingly the name Shoulder Stand. I she needs assistance, he can destroy upon her bottom to move her weight to her shoulders.

Side Saddle

The Side Saddle gives the man a little rest and relaxation while his female partner does all the work. He lies back on the bed, head propped up on a pad, legs outstretched. His female partner squats down on his lap, her feet at his correct thigh. After penetration, she leans back, placing her hands on the bed beside his left thigh. She utilizes her arms for balance and leverage and her legs to move her hips all over while he utilizes his free hands for a little play.

Sidekick

There are sexual positions that give her a brief period to rest and others that give him a brief period to rest – the Sidekick gives the two partners a little rest time. The female lies on the bed on her stomach. She pulls up one knee somewhat and places one arm above her head or under her head. It almost looks as on the off chance that she is falling asleep. Her partner places one knee between her legs and the other on the outside of the outstretched leg. He clutches her back and hip and penetrates from behind.

Sideways Samba

On the off chance that you are ready to add a little dance to your bedroom activities, attempt the Sideways Samba. The female lies on her side, legs outstretched. At the point when outstretched, her body is shaped at a 90-degree angle. He lies beside her as if trying to spoon, yet this position is just temporary. After entering her from the spooning position, he rolls somewhat, lifting his weight with his forearms. He is presently hovering over her bent body penetrating from the top.

Slide

The Slide is a basic yet viable sexual position. The male partner lays flat on his back with his legs loosened up and thighs pressed together. The female partner pays on top of him with her legs loosen up over his. She can wrap her hands around his neck and slide her body here and there for optimal penetration. A few couples find penetration from the final position troublesome so the female partner can straddle the male for penetration before lying down on his chest and outstretching her legs.

Slip

The Slip is a fun, yet somewhat complicated position. The female lies on her back, head on a pad, however back flat on the bed. She twists her knees and pulls her advantages, spreading the legs enough to allow her partner to approach from the front. He slides in the middle of her legs as she lifts her bottom, allowing his knees to slide under. In the event that penetration is troublesome, the male can place his hands under his partner's bottom to lift somewhat and move in nearer.

Snail

During the Snail, the female lies on her back, pulling her knees in toward her chest while lifting her feet off the bed. Her male partner approaches from the front on his knees. As he leans in, placing his hands on either side of her shoulders, she places her feet on his shoulders. Her bottom ought to be lifted off the bed allowing for more profound penetration. Lubrication may be required for the Snail to forestall pain.

Sphinx

The Sphinx is one of only a handful of hardly any belly positions in the Kamasutra. The female lies on her belly. She lifts her chest area somewhat, pulling her forearms under her to hold the majority of her weight. She twists one advantage, pulling her knee in toward her body. The other leg remains loosened up. The male partner approaches from behind, placing one hand on either side of her hips. He enters from this position, his body positioned on the inside of her outstretched leg.

Splitting Bamboo

To perform the Splitting Bamboo, the female lies on her back with her weight moved somewhat to one hip. She lifts the leg on the non-weight bearing side into the air. The male straddles the leg left on the bed and places the lifted leg on his shoulder. The correct leg is placed on the male's left shoulder and the other way around. From this position, the man penetrates and controls musicality. The female can decide to grab his hip, place her hands behind her head, or find another utilization for her free hands.

Squat Balance

The female partner stands on a low table like an end table or coffee table for the Squat Balance. She stands facing away from her partner, who's standing on the floor. He approaches her from behind, yet stops barely shy of penetration. She squats down to sit on his penis. The male partner must support his partner's weight by placing his hands under her bottom. She can reach back and clutch his arms for additional support.

Stairmaster

Have a staircase in your home – why not attempt the Stairmaster? The female partner squats down somewhat on one stair, leans forward, placing her knees on the following stair up and finishes the bow by placing her hands on the following stair (three stairs are involved). It is ideal for picking the stairs nearest the landing to decrease the danger of falling down the stairs. He approaches from behind, placing his knees on the stair where her feet are located. He grabs her hips, enters from behind, and utilizes the hip hold as leverage.

Standing Wheelbarrow

The Standing Wheelbarrow is a gifted sexual position that should just be attempted by solid partners, literally. The female starts the position with knees and hands on the floor (in a Doggy Style position). A pad is placed under her forearms for comfort. Her male partner approaches from behind, kneeling somewhat. He grasps her legs at the ankle, lifting them marginally off the ground (her legs remain bent at the knee) as he penetrated from behind. He should balance her body and control development at the same time.

Star

The Star is similar to the Cross, yet with a wind. The female lies back on the bed with one leg outstretched and the other bent at the knee. Her partner straddles the outstretched leg and tenderly bumps one knee under his partner's bottom (as an afterthought with the bent knee). He leans back, holding his body weight on his arms placed behind him. The male controls penetration; however, the female is allowed to pleasure her or simply appreciate the position.

Creepy crawly

The Spider is one of those positions couples often unearth while transitioning, starting with one position then onto the next. The male is sitting on the bed. His legs are loosened up before him. His female partner sits on his lap, allowing the penis to penetrate. One of her legs is placed on either side of his chest, knees bent. She leans nearly all of her body weight back onto her hands, placed on either side of his legs. She shakes her pelvis to and fro until the two partners climax.

Too 8 / Super 8

The Super 8 is a derivation on the Missionary position. The female lies back on the bed, legs spread apart sufficiently far to allow her partner to move in for penetration. Her feet remain on the bed during the Super 8. The male rests on top of his partner, holding his weight on his outstretched arms. She lifts her hips to meet his cadence. A few ladies find placing a cushion under the bottom makes this position more enjoyable and comfortable.

Supernova

The Supernova is amazing and troublesome at the same time. The male lies on the bed with his head near the foot of the bed. She straddles him in a squat position for penetration. She leans her weight back onto her arms and continues until he is ready to climax. Just before the climax, she drops down to her knees, inches his body off the bed, so his head, chest, and torso are leaning backward – head resting on the floor. She comes back to the squatted, leaning position where she rides until he reaches climax.

Suspended Congress

Hollywood is famous for the Suspended Congress position. The man and the woman will facing each other. His back is near the wall for support. He twists down and lifts her up to a standing sexual position. After penetration, she squeezes her feet against the wall, he lies back onto the wall, and he supports her body weight by placing his hands under her bottom. He controls most development and penetration. However, she can utilize her feet to ricochet.

Suspended Scissors

The Suspended Scissors is an advanced sexual position that requires quality and adaptability with respect to the two partners — the female lies on the bed. Just the lower portion of her body actually on the bed. Her left arm holds her chest area suspended in the air. Her partner then strides through her legs, straddling the leg nearest to the floor. He clutches her other leg with one arm and her waist with the other, creating the scissor reference.

Visitor

The Visitor, another standing position, looks more like a romantic embrace than a sexual position. Male and female stand facing each other, her arms wrapped around his back, and his hands are holding on to her hips and bottom. After using his penis to stimulate her individual, he enters from the front. She can lift her leg marginally to the outside of his thigh to ease penetration. On the off chance that the female partner is significantly shorter than her male partner, she can stand on a stool to make penetration easier.

Whisper

The Whisper looks significantly harder than it actually is. The female lies on her side, pulling the two knees in toward her chest. Her male partner lies on his side, facing her with legs outstretched. She lifts the knee furthest away from the bed far enough to allow him to slide in the middle of her legs and penetrate. She wraps her leg around his body while he pulls her nearby with each push. His weight ought to be somewhat raised as he props his chest area onto his elbow on the bed. She can utilize her free hands to explore.

Widely Open

The Widely Open requires a touch of male chest area solidarity to hold for any time span. The female lies on the bed; a pad is propped under her head. She lifts her knees toward her chest, somewhat lifting her bottom off the bed. Her partner is one of his knees when he approaches her. He slides between her legs, plunks down alone ankles, and penetrates from this seated position. The chest area quality comes in as he places his hands under her back, lifting her body up and toward him in a thrusting movement.

X Rated

The X rated sex position requires control and patience. The male partner lays face up on the bed. The female partner straddles her partner with her back to his face. She brings down her hips for penetration. After penetration, she brings down her chest area between his legs and expands her own legs out straight. Her legs and his legs create the letter X. She slides her body and forward and backward, all over. For added leverage, she can clutch his legs or feet.

Y Curve

The Y Curve requires some solid abdominal muscles and the ideal bed stature. The female lies on her belly. She hurries her body forward until her chest area is bent over the bed – her head resting on her forearms on the floor. His male partner approaches from behind, places his hands on her bottom, and presses up in a cobra yoga position. His legs are loosening up behind him, and he is pushing his chest area up with his arms. His hands are on her bottom, which he utilizes for leverage and development.

Crab's position

The Kama Sutra describes the crab's position as "when both of the legs of the female partner are contracted and place on her stomach." This pose is also known as the intact position. Start with the open-legged position, move on to yawning position and finish with the bent-leg position. The dominance of the man's role makes the pose perfect, especially when he wants to get a little bit rough and spice things up.

From the yawning position, hold your partner's hands so she can't move freely. This will be act as a signal that you want to move into more bondage action. If she is comfortable with it, she can bring her legs close to her body and adopt the submissive crab's position. If she is uncomfortable, don't force it.

Start slowly. When performing the crab's position for the first time, some women may feel that the penetration is too deep. Hold and caress one another's legs and bring your movements in tune as well as make penetration even deeper. Press your chest really close to her shins and make the most of the accessibility of her breasts.

Use your body weight and increase the intensity of the experience, but careful not to press down on her too hard. If needed, use a pillow and make sure your lover's back isn't under any strain. When she is fully aroused, all areas around the pelvis, especially the buttocks and thighs fill with sexual tension. If you want to build the sexual tension up to the screaming point, the crab's position is perfect. Don't penetrate and tease her until she is asking for it. Use your penis and rub it against her clitoris and the insides of her thighs to really turn her on. If your lover still not aroused enough, told her to stay in this position and perform oral sex. This experience will be even more mind-blowing if her legs held firmly in place. When she is completely aroused, move back into position and start the penetration process.

From the woman's viewpoint: don't let him feel he is doing all the work, keep touching him stroke his ears, neck, face, forearms, biceps and anything else within your reach. If you are not comfortable with submissive position, tell him how slow or fast you want him to move.

Lotus-like position

The Kama Sutra says "the Lotus-like position is when the shanks are placed one upon the other". This position is different from the crab's position because you have to cross your shins as if you are meditating sitting cross-legged. Moving into this pose causes the hips to turn outwards and jutting your pelvis out at a slightly changed angle. Some women may feel more comfortable in louts-like position rather than the crab's position, as it gives her more leverage to support her partner's weight. It also allows her to start regaining some of the control.

You need to be extremely supple to adopt this pose. Kneel and support yourself and place a pillow or cushion underneath her to support her weight, as this position will put strain on the shoulder and the neck. Use your hand and move her buttocks to set her pelvis in the best position for both of you. Keep your penis inside her and stimulate her clitoris and anus with your fingers. This position is a natural movement from the crab's position and you don't have to move away from your lover while changing from one pose to another.

Refined position

The pressed positions require strong leg muscles and a lot of stamina. The refine position maintains the excitement, while offer time out from more demanding positions. This can be a welcome progression for the women because in this position she continues to gain more control. This position gives the women the chance to move her legs and change the angle of her pelvis, which means penetration can be more varied and deeper and more mutually satisfying.

From the woman's viewpoint: he keeps his hands on your buttocks and supports your weight. Your legs are around his waist so change the angle and length of penetration if you wish. Tense your thighs and tilt your pelvis up and down to bring you even closer to his genitals. Squeeze the vaginal muscles and grip his penis tighter. The chance for self-stimulation of the breasts means both partners are kept happy.

Half-pressed position

According to the Kama Sutra,"From the pressed position only one of the legs is stretched out, it's called the half-pressed position". This is good for a woman who wants to avoid deep penetration and exercise more control. The woman can vary the sensation by changing the legs, as if you are bicycling with your man and keeping him between your things. You can bend one leg over your partner's shoulder and stretch out the other leg and alternate the pose.

Pressed position

This position is for the couples who like deep penetration. You can easily maneuver your partner into the right position and she keeps firm contact with your body with her feet and hands. Protect her back by supporting her spine with a pillow or with your thighs. This is the ideal pose for men who get really turned on by the sight of their lover's buttocks. Cress the areas around her perineum, anus and inner thighs and increase her arousal.

Before entering your partner, tantalize her by rubbing your penis against the outside of her vagina, buttocks and clitoris. When you are in the throes of lovemaking, add a bit more spice to this position by gently raising her buttocks to make her back rounds.

Hold your partner's ankles and transfer her legs from the side of the center of your body, then down to the other side of the body. Press her feet and clasp her ankles before starting again in the opposite direction. Vary the moves by extending or slowly bending her legs and make sure her vaginal muscles contract around your penis. According to reflexologists, pressing against your partners Achilles'tendon at the heel stimulate the pelvic region even more. With increased arousal, the action can become more vigorous. If she likes a little rough, this will make her crazy. The side position offers an erotic view of her breasts and the intense twisting motion will bring you both a memorable orgasm.

CURIOUS LOVERS

These exciting moves are wonderful for those who are curious but don't want to venture into the land of downright freaky. Each move here will help spice up your bedroom life and try something new, and relatively simple. You will have a wonderful time trying these fabulous positions with your partner, and enhancing your sexy time together. We guarantee you will enjoy these fantastic moves.

THE SPIDER

This position is excellent for long, slow intercourse that enables you to reach orgasm, but not too quickly. It is a unique one that feels great for her, though it may take some effort to get the hang of it. Start by having both the gentleman and the lady laying on their backs with their knees up and slightly spread apart. Then, she should scooch in close to him, and put her legs between his, with her feet up over his hips and next to them. His legs should be under hers, and next to her hips, as well. Then, he can penetrate her and they can gently rock together to achieve the desired depth and rhythm.

CORRIDOR CANOODLING

This is an excellent spur-of-the-moment type position that enables deep penetration. It does, also, require some strength for the gentleman, as he will be performing something similar to a wall sit. It starts by having him in the hallway ("corridor"), in a comfortable wall sit position that isn't too deep. Then, she should have one leg on either side of his legs and sit on his lap. If he is strong enough, she can lift her feet off the floor and he can control the thrusting. If not, she can keep her feet on the ground and the two can work together to control the thrusting, depth, and rhythm.

GALLOPING HORSE

The galloping horse is an exciting, fast-paced position that allows for incredibly deep penetration. The lady has little to no control in this position, which can add to her pleasure. It requires a chair, as other seat choices will not enable the position to work properly. To start, have the gentleman sitting down with his legs straightened and feet on the floor. Then, the lady should sit on his lap, facing him, with a leg on either side. He can then enter her, while she picks her feet up off of the floor and puts them straight out behind him. He can hold her upper arms or shoulders to stop her from falling back, while also giving him leverage to thrust underneath her while she bounces on top of him. It is guaranteed to provide the ultimate deep penetration experience that will send both of you over the edge in no time.

THE GOOD SPREAD

This position is best if the lady is flexible, as it requires her to have her legs stretched out straight to either side. It allows for deep penetration, and for the woman to control the speed and rhythm, as well as where she is being stimulated by him. The man will have free hands, so he can rub her thighs or massage her breasts while she rides him. To start, the gentleman should be lying on his back with his legs however he feels are most comfortable. Then, the lady should mount him, facing him, but sitting upright. Each leg should be stretched out on either side of him, and she can lean forward slightly and use his chest to help her bounce up and down on him. Take care not to bounce out of control, as that could hurt him. Then, he can admire her while she pleasures herself on him.

THE MELODY MAKER

This position takes control away from the female entirely and gives it to the male. It is perfect for hitting the g-spot, and gives the gentleman the ability to use his spare hand to stimulate her clitoris at the same time, ensuring she will achieve a mind-blowing orgasm. Bonus points if they both orgasm at the same time! To start, have the female lay back over a piece of furniture, with her feet firmly on the floor. Then, he can come in between her legs and penetrate her. Depending on the height of the furniture, he may or may not have to get down on his knees to be at the same height as her. He can hold her hands, stimulate her clitoris, massage her breasts, or do anything they desire.

HIT THE SPOT

This position is an excellent behind-entry position that allows for deep penetration and ample stimulation. It might look a bit acrobatic, but it is fantastic for both lovers' pleasure. It is a man-on-top position that almost completely eliminates any control from the female. To start, the lady should be on her tummy on a flat surface. Then, the gentleman should come behind her on his knees, and slide his knees under her tummy. He can enter her similar to doggy-style, while she then wraps one of her legs around him so he can get deeper. He can put his arms next to her and use them to keep her in place.

DASHING RIDER

This is a phenomenal woman-on-top position that can be altered to suit any rider. To start, you want to have the gentleman laying comfortably on his back. Then, the lady can sit on top of him, sideways. She can choose how he penetrates her, and she can ride him at her own chosen speed and rhythm. It helps her control where she is being stimulated and how. It is an easy position that has minimum stimulation over the clitoris and g-spot, but due to the angle makes it feel like she is getting filled completely full.

CAROUSEL

The sex carousel is one of the best positions to achieve deep penetration. It works by having both the lady and the gentleman laying on their backs on the bed, head-to-toe. Then, they should both rise up on their elbows. From there, the lady should put her knees up and her feet over his thighs and up next to his chest. The gentleman can then enter her from beneath, while he wraps one leg up and over her tummy. This gives him leverage to deeply penetrate her and both can achieve an explosive orgasm.

LEGS UP

This position is an awesome one that allows for maximum g-spot stimulation, as well as deep penetration. It is a bit of an experimental position that requires both lovers to practice a little in order to get it perfect, but once it is mastered it can quickly become a favorite position. To start, have the gentleman sit on the floor with his knees bent and legs spread. Then, the lady should sit on the floor in front of him, with her feet up on her shoulders, and her hands on the floor holding her up. He can then thrust from beneath, while she rides him on top. The depth of penetration creates amazing sensations that both will derive pleasure from.

EDGE OF HEAVEN

The edge of heaven positions uses a chair, bed or couch to create heaven's edge. This is an excellent position for the female orgasm, as it creates deep penetration and she is mainly being supported by her sensual areas. To start, the gentleman should sit on the edge of a seat with his feet on the floor. Then, the lady should straddle on top of him on his lap, with a leg on either side of him. The gentleman should then hold underneath her knees, while keeping her legs up in the air, and the lady can balance herself on his lap. He can now thrust as deep and quick as he desires, while stimulating her g-spot and driving her to an incredible orgasm.

MAGIC BULLET

This position is another phenomenal one for deep penetration, and stimulating the g-spot. It is a man-dominant position that is excellent for her pleasure and orgasm. It starts by having the lady laying on her back on the bed. She can either support her head with the bed, or hang her head over the edge of the bed. Then, the gentleman can sit on his knees, spread them wide open, and scooch in close so he can penetrate her. She can put her legs straight up in the air, so the backs of her legs rest on his chest, and he can use her legs for leverage to thrust. For added pleasure and stimulation, she can rub her clitoris to help her achieve orgasm.

Chapter 9 Some Helpful Exercises

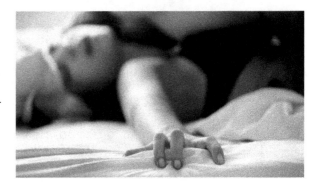

Who doesn't love a good orgasm? There's nothing quite like it. We all seek them out and when we find them, are lost to world - briefly. That said, the other type of orgasm – cosmic, rolling and long lasting – implicates all that we are and for extended periods of time. There is only one way to arrive at this state of bliss and that is through the pursuit of sexual continence. While this may not be for everyone, it's certainly worth a look. Most of us, I'm sure, will be content with re-lighting the flame of passion with our beloved partners. Some of us, though, once that's occurred, will want to take that passion to the next level, which is more intensely spiritual than any other we've discussed. This level of union is the purest form of worship that can be engaged in. Two bodies joined in sexual union, which doesn't have orgasm as its goal, are experiencing a rare state of extended and limitless bliss few others can attain to. For that reason, I'm including this section on supportive exercises for those of you interested in exploring sexual continence and giving it a place in your sacred sexual practice.

Breathing

Improper breathing represents a disconnect between our bodies and our minds. That's because breathing is something we don't think about. It's an automatic, physical function that we do even in the deepest levels of sleep. Breathing mindfully connects our bodies with our minds and opens our awareness to physical sensation. During sexual encounters, particularly when we're seeking to delay orgasm in the service of reaching toward the divine, breathing is a way for us to control the effect of sensation on our orgasmic potential.

There are two principle methods of breathing that can be helpful in this respect. The first is breathing through the nose. Slow, calm breathing, inhaling and exhaling exclusively through the nostrils, is capable of producing a calm, meditative state and sharpening our intellectual connection with the senses, as we experience them. Your metabolic rate, when using this type of breathing, will also be slowed down.

Breathing through the mouth is a natural way of breathing and usually occurs when our bodies demand more oxygen, or when we're expressing an emotion like surprise, or even sorrow. You'll note that when people cry, the mouth is usually open, especially when crying descends into sobbing.

Breathing slowly and mindfully, exhaling and inhaling only through the mouth, also helps the body to release accumulated toxins and helps to relieve tension in the nervous system. Slowing the breathing allows for the body and mind to be integrated in purpose. By briefly holding the breath following inhalation, consciousness is expanded to encompass sensation.

These two basic types of breathing should be practiced with an eye to making them seem more natural. In this way, employing them as part of your sacred sexual ritual will be less forced and much more part of what your living as you enjoy your partner in divine sexual union. Perfecting these before trying the technique I'm about to describe to you is highly recommended.

Breathing deeply is also a way of reducing the influence of stress in your life. As most of us have figured out, stress can put a damper on sex. If we're so exhausted by the endless challenges of everyday living, by the time we've come home to our beloved, how are we to even think about engaging in satisfying, transcendent sex? Getting the stress in our lives under control should be part of our breathing practice and one of the many benefits intentionally-practiced breathing offers.

During sex, depending on your level of mastery over your breathing, the most important thing you can do is to be aware of how you're breathing. Shallow or sharp breaths in the heat of the moment may be unavoidable, to a point. But if you're practicing sexual continence, then it's important both partners be fully aware of the quality of their breathing. Monitoring it and ensuring that your breathing is even and slow helps keep your body relaxed. It also ensures that oxygen is being delivered efficiently and filling your blood cells. This keeps you alive to the moment and focused on what you're doing, which assists you to engage the fullness of your sensuality in your ritual sexual practice.

Re-birthing breathing

This technique's intent is take us back to the first breath we ever drew – the one directly following our arrival on earth. By returning us to that moment, we can experience ourselves on an entirely different level, much more in tune with the cosmos. This method is part of re-connecting with ourselves at the very deepest level.

Lying on your back, with your mouth open, begin to breathe through the mouth, slowly and naturally. Don't force yourself to breathe in any particular way. Just open your mouth and intentionally inhale and exhale through it. Now fill your lungs with air by slowly inhaling. When you're ready to exhale, you'll feel your abdomen deflating naturally.

As you're performing this breathing exercise, think of breathing with your entire body. Intellectually connect those areas of your body you don't normally associate with breathing into the action of your exhalations and inhalations. Visualize your entire body being filled with air, as you slowly inhale and exhale. You will, if you proceed with consistency, take note of a variety of sensations in your body, including tingling. These are due to the influx of oxygen into your system provoked by slow and steady breathing. You will also notice, as you proceed, that your breathing with gradually slow even further. You may sense that you are drifting into a somewhat altered state of consciousness (at least, I hope you do).

It's in this altered state, that you'll be able to experience your body and mind from another perspective. You may find that you're able to visualize yourself in the womb, or in another place from the one you're in (astral projection). What you experience with this exercise is the nature of the universe itself, which is a state of tension holding it together. The tension between opposites (as expressed in the co-creative, sacred sex act) is the glue in the universal structure and is also expressed as the simultaneous expansion and contraction of all that is. This is embodied in your breathing. By fully (but naturally) expelling the air from your lungs in this breathing technique, you are both calling on the past (which is present) and pushing it from you, as you breathe. As you pull air into your lungs, you are pulling the change you desire to know in yourself, inside you, distributing it throughout your body. This plays out as a means of becoming the arya you seek to be.

As you breathe, your intellect and your body will work together to identify points at which you've become blocked, or stuck. This will allow you the opportunity to address these threats to your continuing growth. You may also, with practice, arrive at the point at which you perceive absolutely nothing, and have no discernable thoughts and no consciousness. This is the most desired state achievable, using the re-birthing breathing exercise – that of non-being. Only in this state is true revelation of the self possible, for just beyond it is a place that represents the boundary between our perceptions of life and reality and the truth. That truth is something completely "other"; something that we can't experience in consciousness. In reaching this place, the ecstasy of the truth will open the door to your deepest self-revelation and profound changes that will continue to affect you, long after the breathing exercise has been completed. You will take those changes into the practice of your sacred sexuality and share them with your partner.

In Kama Sutra, sex partners share with one another a divine experience of give and take. This reciprocity should, of course, extend to these breathing exercises. Your partner should also be practicing them.

Exercises to increase male orgasmic control

The first of these is a very simple technique that doesn't require a great deal of explanation, or much imagination to understand. To illustrate, imagine (if you're a male reader) that you're at the proctologist's office. As you assume the position, you hear the familiar, rubberized "snap" behind you, as the good doctor dons his surgical gloves. You know his next move is to insert his finger in a place you'd rather he didn't.

Most male readers will have experienced a pronounced contraction of their anal sphincters as they read the foregoing account. This is a natural, defensive response at the prospect of a foreign object (the proctologist's probing finger), being inserted in the anus. But if you practice this movement regularly, consciously and gradually increase the duration of anal contractions as you grow stronger, you will soon be able to control ejaculation during intercourse. The contraction of the anal sphincter serves the purpose of preventing orgasm from occurring before you want it to. This is an easy method, but one that takes a little time, patience and practice. Starting with 30 repetitions, you'll soon find that the contraction of these muscles is easy and takes very little effort on your part.

Another technique involves the small area between the male testicles and the anus. This area, when pressed, inhibits the ability of sperm to flow to the shaft of the lingam and then, be ejaculated. Placing a finger on this spot and applying pressure at the right moment will stop ejaculation from occurring.

Finally, squeezing the shaft of the yoni, when the male senses ejaculation is imminent, can serve to stop climax from occurring. Firmly gripping and then squeezing the shaft works as a way of distracting the mind from the impending orgasm, allowing the man to continue with sex by delaying it.

Sexual continence is a much more achievable goal for women. Generally speaking, orgasm is more of a long term project for women and thus, not the great issue it is for men. The male climax can arrive at inopportune moments; moments at the woman partner is far from happy with her experience. This is an impediment to arriving at the divine state of sexual union that eludes so many of us.

Despite the more time-consuming nature of female orgasm, it's also advisable that women use the breathing exercises outlined in this section. Delaying their own orgasms can lead to the type of cosmic orgasm I've described elsewhere in this book. Learning to breathe slowly and intentionally and live in the sexual moment is not just for men. It's for women, too. You're both in this together and a little solidarity, as the male partner seeks to delay his orgasm, can be a strong binding agent and yet another way to increase the sexual bond between you.

Kegels – strengthening the Yoni

Many women today practice Kegel exercises. These can serve to help women regain the yoni's natural elasticity, following childbirth, as well as restore their ability to retain urine for long periods of time (which can be effected by childbirth, also). For those of you reading though, Kegel exercises are a way to strengthen the muscles of the yoni, in order to be able to use them as a way to increase both your pleasure and that of your partner.

The muscles engaged when using Kegel exercises are those located in the pelvic floor. If readers are unsure as to where they are and how to "flex" them, they can find them by stopping the flow of urine the next time they visit the washroom. The muscles that stop the flow are those we're looking for. Women readers can practice doing this several times, until they can engage these muscles when they're not urinating. Also, Kegel exercises shouldn't be used to stop the flow of urine as a habit. This can lead to the bladder getting the message that it should retain some of the urine it needs to eliminate and can result in bladder infections, which most will agree are very unpleasant.

Kegel exercises, practiced as a series of contractions and releases can be started by holding the engagement of these pelvic floor muscles for a count of five. A good place to start is with a set of ten of these. Once readers feel they've mastered this stage of development, they can move on to ten sets of ten count contractions, resting for ten seconds between each. Making a habit of doing these exercises every day, will result in readers having the ability to amaze their partners with their superior muscle control. Male partners may be screaming for mercy, once their women have Kegeled their way to stronger yonis!

Exercise for better sex

Some will not much care to hear this, but it needs to be said. Physical fitness makes sex a lot more fun. Especially if you're planning on practicing sexual continence for prolonged love making, the last thing you want is to get tuckered out before you've gotten anywhere near that sexual ecstasy you're hoping for.

Of particular importance is cardiovascular health. We've all heard stories of people who've suffered cardiac events in the throes of passion. If you're concerned that might end up being you, then it's time to take the bull by the horns and treat your heart to more of what it needs – exercise. All exertion will become easier for you and your sexual encounters will be effortless, when you're not concerned that your heart may not be meeting the challenge.

Walking regularly is a pleasant and healthy way to get more exercise and it's also an enjoyable activity you can do with the god or goddess in your life, as you plan your new life of sexual connection and fulfilment. You don't have to run a marathon. You don't have to scale Everest. You just need to feel your best, because part of being the best possible version of yourself is your wellness. You and your partner will thank me later, even if the thought of exercise leaves you cold now.

Another extremely effective form of exercise is planking (which comes to us from the world yoga, discussed below). While some of you may believe this is too challenging, planking is achievable for people of almost every fitness level. It is a silver bullet that engages a broad array of the body's muscle groups. Start by holding the plank for ten seconds, adding additional time as you're able. Soon you'll find that your posture and muscle tone have improved dramatically, as you're able to hold the plank for longer periods of time. There is also a strong meditative aspect to the plank, when held for longer duration. This type of focus will serve you well, as you seek the divine in your sex life, together.

If you're not sure how to properly execute a plank, be sure to explore online resources, or consult with a fitness professional in your area. Planking, in only a few minutes every day, can make you much stronger and more physically ready to enter into a world of erotic delight with your partner.

Yoga

Yoga is a natural ally of those who are undertaking the spiritualization of their sexuality. Yoga can help prepare your bodies for the sexual journey you're embarking on by attuning it to the project.

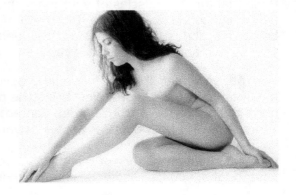

Chapter 9 Some Helpful Exercises | 75

Yoga incorporates its own type of breath control, which is called "pranayama". This type of breathing is responsible for releasing oxytocin into the blood stream, which enhances the sex drive (see further on in this section for more on pranayama). An added benefit is improved flow of blood to your genitals, which adds to the effect of the breathing techniques involve. Yoga has also been proven to help men achieve erections of longer duration and increased testosterone production. Following are some simple poses to begin with, which are specifically geared to improving stamina and strength for more effortless sex. Perhaps you'll find you enjoy yoga and want to go further with your practice. In that case, there's no shortage of yoga studios just about anywhere the world you can think of, as yoga has become the aerobics of the 21st Century.

The Chair

This pose is particularly useful for women, as it engages the muscles of the pelvic floor in the same way the Kegel exercises do (see above in this section). The practice of this pose, then, is a good compliment to women using the Kegel to strengthen their yonis' ability to grip the male lingam.

As you perform this pose, pretend you're about to sit in a chair. Stand with your feet together and touching. Now, bend your knees as you would to become seated in a chair, bent slightly forward from the waist. Raise your arms over your head, relaxed, but elongated. Now consciously elongate the lowest part of your spine (tailbone/coccyx). By engaging the muscles in your pelvic floor, this part of your spine will be pulled back and straightened, aligning your upper body. Make sure to engage your abdomen and back muscles. Hold for as long as you're comfortable with. As you become stronger, you'll be able to hold this and other poses longer.

The Squat

This pose is exactly what it sounds like. You will perform a deep squat. Beneficial for the muscles of your inner thighs, the squat also engages the pelvis and serves to promote the health of all the joints in this region of the body. Your abdominal muscles are also engaged. It's believed by some that your spleen and reproductive system are stimulated by this pose, also.

With your feet apart at just a little beyond the width of your hips, your toes should be turned out. Now bring the palms of your hands together and place them directly in front of you, centered over the chest area. Now lower yourself toward the floor. Get as low as you can, comfortably, without straining yourself. Keeping your spine long and engaging your abdominal muscles will yield the greatest benefit of this pose. If you're able and wish to stretch your inner thighs, you can use your elbows to push your knees out further.

The squat can also be performed with the feet wide apart (toes still pointed out). This is probably the more realistic option for beginners, as it's somewhat less demanding. In this variation, lower yourself to the level of your knees, with your arms up and bent at the elbow, palms facing forward.

The Cobra

This well-known yoga pose is an excellent stretch for the abdominal muscles and for the associated muscle group that extends into the genital region and the pelvis. This is an excellent pose couples can engage in immediately before a session of prolonged sex.

Lying on your stomach with your legs together, push yourself up with your palms flat to support the weight of your upper body. Make sure to engage your abdominal muscles when you do this, in order to protect your back. If you're a beginner, keep the neck long and the head facing forward, as you imagine pressing your pelvis into the floor. Once you've become accustomed to this pose, you can pull your head back to look up, taking great care not to strain your neck and remembering to hold your shoulders down (don't let them drift up to your ears, as this aspect of the pose strengthens the arms, shoulders and upper back).

If you find this classical version of the cobra too difficult, you can raise yourself on your elbows, with your forearms extended in front of you. This will not achieve the deep stretch of the classic, but it's safer if it's been awhile since you engaged in any type of deep stretching activity. Safety first! It's difficult to engage in prolonged lovemaking when your neck is out!

Pranayama breathing

In Sanskrit, "prana" means "life force". By learning to breathe in a way that allows the life force to flow through you unobstructed, you are releasing its power. A fitting introduction to this type of breathing is the "Challenger" (known in Sanskrit as "ujjayi pranayama", which means "hissing breath"). Let's review how it's accomplished, step by step.

This style of pranayama produces a gentle hiss, as the breath is drawn in and out, over the posterior section of the throat. This may sound difficult, but if you practice it mindfully and intentionally, you'll learn how to do it.

Seat yourself in the lotus position (or modified lotus, if you find the classic version uncomfortable). You can also seat yourself in a chair, with your back straight and your shoulders relaxed. Both feet should be flat on the floor, if seated. Your hands may be placed in your lap, the right hand over the left, palms up and thumbs touching.

Draw your breath in through your nose, exhaling through your open mouth. As you breathe in an out, consciously seek to draw your breath across the back of your throat. For the exhale, accompany it with a protracted "ha". After repeating your exhalation and inhalation a few times, close your mouth. You're now going to do the same, using your nose for both inhalations and exhalations.

As you inhale and exhale, visualize your breath flowing across the back of the throat. As you do this, you should be hearing a gentle hissing (for which this type of pranayama is named). This is known as the "unspoken mantra" and its benefits are threefold. Your breathing will become slower. The sound also helps your mind to focus on your breathing and prevent it from adhering to stray thoughts that may distract you. As you monitor the hissing sound, ensuring that it maintains the same quality from beginning to end of your breaths, your flow is naturally rendered more smooth.

Practicing the challenger style of breathing can begin with a five to eight-minute session, which you may gradually increase to ten and eventually, fifteen minutes. When you've completed your breathing practice, you should revert to breathing as you normally do, still either in the lotus, or seated, for several minutes. Following this, lay down for a little while to return to your normal frame of mind and to absorb what you're feeling as the result of your breathing practice.

With time and dedicated practice, you'll find that the benefits of ujjayi pranayama include quieting your mind, which allows increased focus in every area of life and, of course, in your sexual practice. When both partners practice breathing in this way together, the mutual benefits will soon become apparent in your lovemaking. Synchronizing your breath to one another and using some of the techniques found in this chapter will prove enormously helpful for strengthening your connection with each other and supporting extended love making – especially when sexual continence is being practiced.

Conclusion

As you enhance your sexual repertoire, you'll likely find that the passion you achieve in the bedroom will transcend into other aspects of your life. Couples that are intimate and sexually satisfied tend to have a healthier relationship overall. Of course, don't forget to have fun, and approach the Kama Sutra with a positive attitude, and be open to all of the things that you may discover while exploring your loved one in the most intimate ways possible.

Kama Sutra is a guide book for love and everything involved in loving another person. It is more than just a book of sex positions, but these days most people only know it for its complex and flexibility-requiring positions for intercourse. The book of Kama Sutra includes a general guide to living well in ways other than through sex. It includes a guide to foreplay, a guide to kissing and touching, as well as other ways to achieve intimacy with your partner, such as bathing together and giving each other massages. I hope that after reading this book, you understand and can appreciate this text in a new way.

By opening up this book, you have already taken the first step in preparing yourself for your new sex life. By informing yourself as much as you can, you will ensure you are as prepared as possible so that you will be able to experience as much pleasure as you can. At the end of the day, sex is about pleasure, and knowing how best to please yourself and your sexual partners will keep them coming back to you again and again. You are going to thank yourself for having picked up this book.

In addition to the positions enclosed in these pages, I hope that you learned how to focus on your pleasure and the pleasure of your partner, how to be present during sex, and how to become more sexually intuitive in order to feel the most pleasure possible. What a waste of pleasure it would be to always have sex in the same positions over and over and never fully reach your potential for orgasm! If you haven't already, try some of the things you've learned through reading this book, and I assure you that your sex life will be much better for it!

We do our best to reach out to readers and provide the best value we can. Your positive review will help us achieve that. It'd be highly appreciated!

Printed in the USA
CPSIA information can be obtained
at www.ICGtesting.com
LVHW021039070823
754530LV00020B/230